Light-Bulb Moments

Simulated Patients in East Midlands Healthcare

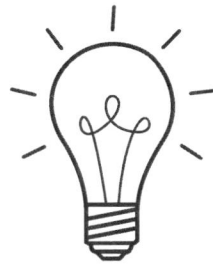

Peter Worrall

Designed by **Sophie Hardwicke**
Illustrations by **Ian Mitchell**
Diagrams by **Chris Cooper-Hayes**

Published by Retep Press
36 West Avenue, Clarendon Park,
Leicester LE2 1TR
March 2014
ISBN 978-0-9927120-0-6
Printed by Rural Press Ltd, Leicester

Contents

Acknowledgements

Ron Thew, in collaboration with his patients Brenda and Richard Smith, quietly developed what later became the Leicester Method for real patient simulation. In similar vein, David Sowden and Justin Allen, having foreseen the educational benefits of developing a team of simulators, quietly provided the necessary professional and financial support.

I cannot reliably list all the simulators and doctors who've been involved in our SP journey. There's a long list of doctors in the South Trent, later LNR Deanery, and Leicester Medical School who've given up time to design or record SP roles and facilitate them with flair. Then, there are the forty or more SPs who've striven to represent the 'patient voice'. Over the years their focus on task, their persistence in adapting to circumstances, combined with their enjoyment in working together, has been a personal delight. Such companionship is rare. I trust they'll all know to whom I refer.

There are two people to whom I owe a particular debt of gratitude:

Gus Gresham, a writer and SP volunteered to read chapters as they emerged – yes, volunteered out of sheer goodwill. As month followed month, I've received and attended to his comments. Not only has he corrected my punctuation, kindly and persistently; even more valuably, he's forced me to be more succinct and reconsider my loosely expressed language.

My debt to Brenda, wife and fellow SP, is immeasurable. Despite having many other interests, she's made typescripts of recordings that now appear as East Midlands SP examples. She's found time to read and comment on first drafts and furthermore, her comments have been ruthlessly constructive – deeply perceptive. I'm truly grateful.

The Author

Peter Worrall taught in and managed schools in the UK and abroad for over 30 years. Conversation with a doctor friend in 1992 led to him becoming a simulated patient and then leader of the Leicester Simulated Patient Unit. His experience includes work as a non-clinical GP course organiser and ten years collaboration with the team that published *Advanced Consulting in Family Medicine: the consultation expertise model* (2009) about the nature of expert GP consultation. He is currently interested in simulating aspects of aging!

Part One
Simulator and Facilitator Expertise

Chapter One

Introduction _____

Light-Bulb Moments

I've chosen the book's title to symbolise what can happen when a group of health professionals come together with a facilitator and simulated patient to explore their own practice. In day-to-day life, light-bulb moments may signify minor insights of the *'oh I get it'*, variety, often kept to ourselves. Whereas, here we are concerned with those more professional moments relevant to doctors, nurses and a wide range of health workers. Dramatic light-bulb moments can impact on all concerned. Here's an illustration from my own experience: it concerns a breaking bad news scenario originally written for GP speciality registrars and acted out in a small training group. In this case Mrs Brownlow is thought to be drinking a bottle of sherry a day and thus in danger of shortening her life.

Mrs Jean Brownlow is 58 and has been a widow for ten years. Her late husband was an accountant who left her with few money worries. She has one daughter and two grandchildren living locally. Her son-in-law is adamantly teetotal. Mrs Brownlow would like to spend time with her grandchildren but is not welcome in their house. She has a history of liver problems and has been told by the hospital that she has pancreatitis. The GP registrars decided it was necessary to confront her drinking. One after the other they tried to find out how much she was drinking by using confrontational medically related questions. Each was rebuffed in a quietly controlled way. Mrs Brownlow's denial seemed to be impregnable.

Then one of the group sat in the consulting chair, paused, and said quietly, 'You must have been very lonely in that big house after your husband died'.

Mrs Brownlow immediately broke down, 'Yes' she said through her tears, 'and I'm so ashamed.

It started because the days were so long with nobody to talk to and then I couldn't stop. I've since had to become clever at hiding the bottles in the compost heap and taking them to the bottle bank after dark'.

Sighs of relief all round. *He's cracked the impasse, now we can talk about her health*. It was an instant light-bulb moment, a breakthrough, an unplanned example of the power of empathy. At a more analytical level, it's an example of patient-centred consulting. The calm, quiet manner and tone of the doctor's voice was also worthy of comment. Furthermore, here was a good example of an 'opportune moment': an unexpected opportunity to make a fundamental learning point. Group work of this kind can evoke many such learning layers as I hope to show.

Keeping the light on

This valuable simulation approach is now being crowded out by a preoccupation with high investment technology, and of course, by constrained budgets. That is not to say there's a conflict between using person-to-person and high-tech approaches: both have virtue. High-tech rightly dominates because it's concerned with patient safety and the facility to train people off the job, particularly in secondary care. That said, there is a sixty-year history of 'live', patient simulation. For the remainder of Light-Bulb Moments the initials SP will be used as will be explained in the next chapter on Clarifications. I can perhaps be forgiven for feeling miffed at the dismissive way it is currently being treated. As an example, the quotation below is the only (inaccurately expressed) mention of simulated patients to be found in an important DoH publication concerned with simulation and e-learning, and that despite a strong emphasis on 'patient centred and service driven' care.

Another widely used form of simulation is the 'simulated patient', where individuals, usually trained actors, mimic patient symptoms and problems to allow exploration of the learner's responses and communication skills in a standardised format. Simulated patients are often used in student and trainee examinations.

A Framework for Technology Enhanced Learning, Department of Health, 2011

The following chapters are written for simulators playing patients and health educators controlling their use. The intention is to illustrate the virtues and practice of quality SP practice, together with stories from a wide range of training applications, in order to keep the light burning.

Contents

Part One of the book is concerned with SP and facilitator practice. It covers group learning processes, interpersonal skill content and feedback outcomes. From the introduction of a novice there's a jump to indications of what highly skilled SPs and facilitators do. This jump, an omission of what might be called the 'experiential journey', is quite deliberate. Detail of how SPs and facilitators can and should work is already available in manuals and other publications. More apposite in our locality is that most SPs and facilitators are left to learn from experience with minimum training and scant access or time to benefit from publications.

To be fair, the training scene is not so dire. There is always specific training when SPs and facilitators are used for the assessment of medical competence; OSCEs (Objective Standardised Clinical Assessments) are used throughout medical schools. Even more exacting for our SPs is the training to participate in the selection assessment for admission to GP speciality training. For this, national assessment criteria govern local selection centres; a rare example of cross country coordination. As an SP group we experienced the previous process first hand when we were engaged with Summative Assessment SP Surgeries. Assessment experience undoubtedly contributes to skill levels. Nevertheless, I've excluded this aspect of work here because of its specificity; I can only write as a practitioner, not as an examiner. Hence the declaration:

The practice of using simulators for assessment is not included as the multiplicity of examining procedures is usually prefaced by specific training.

In similar vein, it should be noted that I've assumed an umbilical link between SPs and facilitators. The interdependence of the two skills is generally assumed but rarely recognised. There is of course a difference in status; SPs as casual labour hardly compare with salaried nurses, doctors and health workers. But, when on task, their skills are of equal importance in terms of the quality of group learning. And experienced SPs do become simulator educators, often switching to facilitation techniques in the same session!

There is a need for simulation and facilitation to be accorded equal importance

Part Two consists of thirteen case stories recounting how facilitators and simulators have been used for healthcare purposes in the East Midlands. Why be so specific you may ask? Surprisingly, given that simulated patients have been involved in medical training since Howard Barrows first introduced them in 1963 and a detailed manual was published by Fiona Dudley in 2012 (The Simulated Patient Handbook), the practice varies considerably from locality to locality. For example, there are medical schools in the Netherlands and USA with impressive premises specifically designed for multiple SP use. There, simulators are recruited in large numbers, initially trained for several days, used extensively for individual student training which is filmed and scrutinised for proficiency of both student and system. They are also used extensively in OSCE assessment. I doubt whether any UK medical school is able to replicate such extensive use of

SPs, for cost, if no other reason.

The case stories I've included illustrate a wide range of SP use: from patients for the development of consulting skill, to trauma victims on a paramedic trolley. Few will be aware of SP inclusion as relatives in a highly complicated workshop to explore the complexities of organ donation. How often, for example, have SPs been involved, not only as key elements in a serious research project, but also in a subsequent workshop for GP practitioners? Most of the other stories relate either to regular training use or innovative activity, with one nearby exception, in the East Midlands, i.e. Leicestershire, Rutland, Nottinghamshire, Derbyshire and for medical purposes Lincolnshire. This prompts another declaration:

Local experience as portrayed here is presented as an opportunity for comparison with other regions and emphatically not as a statement of special value.

Turning experience into expertise

'Being' an authentic patient, doctor, nurse or health worker, at increasing levels of complexity, involves high levels of personal skill that can only grow with experience. Similarly, facilitators require personal skill to manage group learning, whatever the topic and learning level of the group. This also requires a progression of experience. The quality of what happens when those skills are put to use demands knowledge from other than medical disciplines. The iceberg metaphor helps us picture how these skills rely on a wealth of knowledge, if we are to affect others in a way that ensures that learning impacts on clinical expertise.

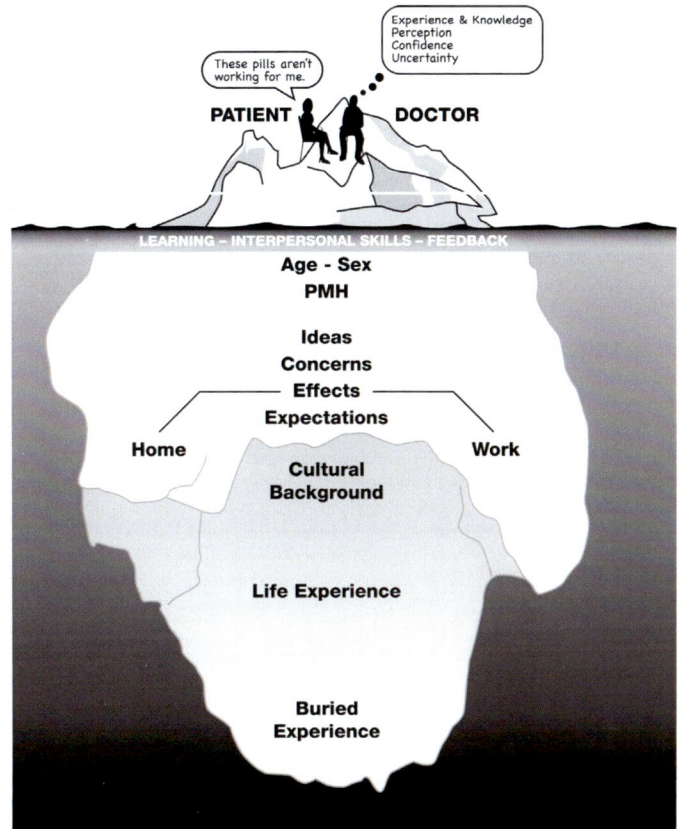

Although simulated patients may be used for a variety of purposes, such as demonstrations before a large audience, their customary use is with small groups of less than ten people. How best to manage groups of disparate learners in varied learning arenas requires specialist knowledge of group and learning processes in order to take people below the water level into those depths and shallows that affect our wellbeing.

What lurks 'below the water line' is often crucial to a diagnosis, and to patient safety and therapeutic care; it's a significantly practical metaphor.

It must be emphasised that there is a clinical context in almost all simulated patient sessions. Evolving Advanced Care Plans with terminally ill patients, one of the stories in Part Two, though heavily socially biased, has a medical sub-text. Clinical content needs to be taken as integral to all activity, but since we are always dealing with unique individuals, interpersonal skill becomes a matter of parallel priority.

When a group member consults with a simulated patient in the company of colleagues there are heightened learning opportunities. And whatever anyone says about the artificiality of simulation, it is very real for those involved. In sensitive hands, what happens will have sharpened learning potential. The person consulting will be behaving in a manner very similar to day to day practice; their level of skill will be exposed for comment – usually in relation to a declared learning purpose. A rich dialogue is possible, BUT, only if what is fed into that dialogue is constructive and immediate. To that end the facilitator's skill in eliciting quality feedback is of major importance.

The three multi-faceted areas of special knowledge on the previous diagram – there below water level to be called upon when appropriate – are vital for the development of expertise. Knowing when and how to call upon them enriches the learning potential as well as adding to the quality of facilitator and simulator expertise. All concerned can learn from the group activity.

The prime purpose of *Light-Bulb Moments* is to encourage the growth of expertise in this important medical learning context.

Content grounded in personal experience

Using local experience has key implications for the Light-Bulb Moments approach. One is that it is inescapably based on personal experience. And two, the way work has emerged locally may well, in retrospect, present a distinctive low cost, low investment model.

Personal background

I became a simulator after a career in education with, I must add, some amateur dramatic experience hidden in the depths of my uncalled-for CV. At the time, I was one of four simulators; the others were a county councillor, a drama teacher and a hospital administrator. That was

20 years ago at a time when a group of local GP educators, then called Course Organisers, met the entire cohort of GP trainee registrars every Wednesday afternoon. The registrars met whether they were on their hospital or GP rotations, i.e. *there was inbuilt experiential continuity.*

By chance, one of the course organisers felt the need to develop patient simulations based, with consent, on videotaped consultations of his patients. This was to become the Leicester Method for role development. By chance again, I happened to know one of the other course organisers through another activity. He was a doctor who foresaw the wider potential and was also, by chance, involved in work for the Royal College of General Practitioners.

As a consequence of local initiatives, end of line budget money, and out of locality connections, a team of simulators emerged. These simulators, encouraged by the mutuality of doctor-simulator activity, gained experience from being involved in consultation skill development across a wide range, i.e. *there was continuity of institutional sponsorship.*

More formative experiences

Because of changes in the assessment of GP certification methodology, we also became involved in the research and eventual establishment of Simulated Patient Surgeries. These surgeries became an authorised alternative to the submission of video tapes for the assessment of consultation skills at national level. As one factor in the certification to practise as a GP, this was a high-stake process. Seasonally, we ran twice weekly simulated surgeries, in which each candidate consulted with eight different patients. As simulators, we were also trained and trusted to mark the clinical checklists and patient rating scales.

A parallel aspect of our work concerned the design of workshops for specific consulting purposes. These joint simulator–doctor presented workshops were regularly booked by other regional GP training schemes. So we became familiar in depth with one area of training and aware of a wide range of simulation uses as shown in the following list.

Examples
Simulation Activities Over the Years

Medical School small group communication skill training and OSCEs

Demonstration of simulation potential at RCGP and WONCA Conference (Dublin).

Consultation skill workshops on ICE, Dealing with Difficult Patients, Breaking Bad News, Dealing with Cultural Diversity, Concordance, Telephone Consulting at GP Vocational Training Schemes throughout the East Midlands and Implications of patient-centred Consulting

Health Which projects to test the effectiveness of private GP drop-in centres in London railway stations, slimming clinics and NHS Direct – also NHS Direct drop-in centres, i.e. as incognito patients

Simulated Patient Surgeries for GP Summative Assessment – annually for seven years. Surgeries of 13 cases seen by one doctor to establish evidence of competence (NCAS)

Various assessment procedures for OSCEs and Royal College purposes

Sessions throughout the country to assist pharmacists practise engaging in more detailed patient consultations

Filmed consultations to establish nature of expert GP consulting, leading to Advanced Consulting in Family Medicine, published in 2009

Trial work for GP Selection Centres and the Therapeutic Rapport model

Practice nurse training assessments ; End of Life training workshops; Doctor appraiser training

Relatives in a variety of secondary care training situations

Our team of simulators expanded along with our range of experience and collective expertise. Meanwhile however, hardly noticed by us simulators, the context was changing. National attention was focused anew on the training and assessment of all doctors. The Royal College of General Practitioners (RCGP) centralised the assessment for college membership in London. So, there were no more simulated patient surgeries run outside London. Although we did some work with nurses, most of what we did was in Primary Care, where major changes were being made to training programmes. Locally this led to fewer course organisers, now renamed programme directors (PDs). Monthly meetings for registrars replaced weekly meetings. The introduction of and preoccupation with the new e-portfolio, work-based assessment, inevitably led to less SP based learning. On reflection, cost implications and increasingly busy training practices may well have further eroded a focus on quality consulting practice, our primary function.

Putting aside political and organisational changes over time, there is a little considered consequence of the local initiative factor so commonly associated with SP practice. Initially there is much enthusiasm and the range of work increases through word of mouth between professional colleagues. But the enthusiasts move to other posts and grow older. So gradually, wider knowledge of SP benefit diminishes and the volume of work declines. The antidote is institutionalisation, as is the case with medical schools.

For administrative reasons, our disparate group of simulators were adopted by a simulation centre in another city – a centre with the full range of up-to-date high tech equipment. The centre was already working to full capacity with its focus in secondary care, so it was an act of charity to accept us lot with our focus in primary care. We were thus introduced to roles that were ancillary to clinical priorities, unlike the interpersonal focus central to consulting in family medicine we'd been accustomed to. For example, becoming a relative alongside a critically ill manikin requires some rethinking of the learning situation you're in. Our range extended over time to include psychiatric patients, doctors, pharmaceutical customers and veterinary clients. Most of this activity depended on the commitment and versatility of the simulators and the level of skill they accrued from experience. The same can be said for facilitators. *Light-Bulb Moments* is designed to reflect and support such a process.

A model approach?

I have referred to our way of working as a '**low-cost self-reliant model**' but that's only a personal opinion. My sole justification is comparison with the impressively elaborate way in which standardised patients are used for undergraduate medical training, as evidenced by Maastricht Medical School and similar practices in the USA. I look forward to being corrected.

Localism

Localism simply reflects the manner in which various health-training agencies work. It is not about narrow mindedness! Indeed, more accurately, it reflects the degree of local initiative in the vastness of health provision. To this may be added the enclosed nature of simulated-patient-based activity. SPs and facilitators are rarely seen by outside observers. As long as sessions end with a general feeling of it having been worthwhile there is a minimum of debriefing and critique. Hanging over the activity is the largely unexplored question of whether sessions do lead to changed behaviour – the question of measurability. So activity does remain largely local with limited inter-regional connection for simulators and facilitators. By contrast, at the health educator level, there are national and international organisations, conferences, academic books and journals and interplay of ideas and practice. Nevertheless, for simulators and facilitators the focus tends to be on the next local session.

The need to provide reliable assessment procedures for the selection of general practice registrars for specialty training is an exception. Much of the initial research that led to the current procedures was conducted in the East Midlands, so we have sense of how this process has developed over time. As with any national assessment procedure there is now an overarching organisation with a duty to provide common practice. The NRA (National Recruitment Agency) has declared that all simulators recruited to this important process should be experienced. Locally, this has not been a problem so far but, if 'live' simulated patient opportunities are crowded out by the dominance of high-tech simulation and cost cutting, this may become the case – just one of the reasons for the publication of *Light-Bulb Moments*.

Expertise development

The emphasis throughout is devoted to the development of expertise from a practitioner point of view. Application of this expertise is primarily focused on learning contexts concerned with patient care and colleague teamwork. Essential to this are the discrete fields of interpersonal skills and 'human factors'; the one mainly concerned with interaction with patients and the other with colleagues. Case stories in Part Two provide examples of both.

In the main, facilitators are engaged from the clinical areas related to the chosen learning purpose. Although there is no chapter exclusively concerned with the various specialised workplaces under consideration, it is vitally important that simulators, as they become more experienced, are not only aware of the different contexts but have some understanding of contextual issues, such as clinical uncertainty or the implications of patient-centred consulting.

There is a need to enhance the profile and revive the value of simulated patients and their facilitators as partners in the wider world of simulation.

Chapter Two
Clarifications

In order to concentrate on day to day practice, unclouded by what is happening in the current world of simulation, it is necessary to start with a working knowledge of the context – the understandings, the issues and the problems of vocabulary.

Simulation in the world at large

Simulation is a technique, not a technology, to replace or amplify real experience with guided experiences often immersive in nature that evoke or replicate substantial aspects of the real world in a fully interactive fashion.

DM Gaba, The Future Vision of Simulation in Healthcare, *Quality and Safety in Healthcare*, 2004

Not so long ago anyone asking, 'What's a simulation?' would have been well served with a dictionary definition. Now the answer must be more elaborate. Indeed simulation seems to be spreading like a hardly noticed virus. My first experience of what I now consider to be a simulation was when it was common for young people and first aiders to be trained in emergency resuscitation with the help of a manufactured body called 'resusci-annie'. You could do all sorts of mischief to 'annie' without hurting anyone. Now we have highly sophisticated manikins that breathe, bleed and can die with dignity.

As a proud parent I once watched my daughter, aged 12, enter a swimming pool in a lifesaving competition. She and her life-saving club team were confronted by a pile of floating junk partly covered with a tarpaulin. What I knew and she didn't was that there was a person underneath the pile who was in danger of drowning. The team was awarded points according to their life-saving techniques and how they worked as a team, i.e. a simulation – a set-up designed to assess knowledge and skill in a practical fun way.

Recently, unknown to its doctors and nurses, a major local hospital trust used this approach on a massive scale to test its emergency capability. Nowadays the army, police, fire brigades and other services routinely create near reality simulations to train their staff for future action in the real world.

In parallel with these very practical and time-hallowed techniques, simulation is now used to replicate reality by means of electronic media or mathematical modelling. Most common of course is its use for computer games. In the technical field new technology has customarily been tried out, revised and tested with mock-ups and models. Simulated car crashes, for example, are used to devise better safety features. Now whole systems, such as new railway projects, can be simulated not only to test an infinite amount of technical and operational detail but to be used subsequently to train operating staff. In Lincoln, at the Institute of Food Research, a model gut is used to 'understand and predict the behaviour of food within a digestive tract, thus permitting well informed interventions to improve health', i.e. simulation assisted research, a more sophisticated form of trial and error!

Without doubt, for me, the most esoteric use of computer simulations is by archaeologists who attempt to predict what might have happened during, for instance, the Neolithic period, as society became less peripatetic; what degree of collaboration was there between settlements, what kind of leadership emerged. More tangible simulations prepare visual representations of what a settlement might have looked like based upon specific excavations and other evidence. Exciting stuff! If I understand it correctly, the term *emergence* is central to this kind of simulation, i.e. what emerges when a set of known variables come together. The unpredictability of what emerges from the interaction in an archaeological simulation can throw up new ideas and concepts that can be checked against the known evidence. Nothing to do with patient simulation you may say. Certainly not! But if you equate the mathematical model with the individual variables of an adult learning group, what *emerges* is comparably unpredictable, and immeasurable. But maybe this is a comparison too far?

According to different dictionaries simulation can involve: imitation or enactment; the act or process of pretending or feigning; an assumption or imitation of a particular appearance or form; counterfeit or sham. So there can be a dark side, as when SPs present as 'incognito patients', as real patients in real situations.

> *'… medical simulation takes advantage of contextual and experiential learning by allowing trainees to practise in realistic environments prior to actual patient care'*
>
> Huang, Gordon and Schwartzstein, Millennium Conference 2005 on Medical Simulation: A Summary Report. *Simulation in Healthcare*, Vol. 2, No 2, 2007

Simulation as used in medicine embraces a full spectrum of simulation resources for the purpose of education and training. **Here there should be no deception.** The artifice should be clear and participants need to become proficient at learning and being assessed by this means. That said, it is imperative that doctors, nurses and others who engage with simulated patients and high-tech simulators <u>must</u> behave as their day-to-day professional selves.

While involved in simulated activities participants must become accustomed to behaving naturally, as themselves, and treat the situation as if it is real

Nomenclature – words used and their meaning

Let's start with the term 'human simulator'. What does that mean? Is it you or me on a bed with a drip attached, or is it the name of the human plastic look-alike that can bleed and pee with a voice that comes from a microphone hidden behind a one-way glass wall? You've guessed – it's the high-priced manikin. Please excuse me if that sounds a bit peevish. After all it is a perfectly correct label; the manikin does simulate a human being and as such is of irreplaceable value in teaching new hospital doctors. The trouble is it leaves me wondering what to call myself; patient simulator – simulated patient? The manikin is both. 'Live' or 'individual' simulator? That doesn't sound right either!

In the USA alternatives to using real patients for training were initiated in the 1960s and called standardised patients. In the UK we've always been referred to as simulated patients without any confusion. This remains sensible as standardisation is a word better reserved for establishing equality of challenge in the world of assessment. I can illustrate the distinction from a regrettable personal experience as an SP.

In an assessment scenario I was the husband in a quandary regarding the outcome of his wife's surgical operation. Subsequent to a request for information required to make family plans that depended on the length of her hospital stay, I was to meet a junior doctor (candidate). Though a member of the department this doctor had not been able to confer with her senior and was thus unable to provide accurate facts – a difficult task to test the doctor's ability to protect the clinical circumstances and mollify me.

I had been suitably trained to present an opening sentence followed by a series of mandatory questions to provide evidence for two observers – a standardised assessment process I'd been through many times. That day, after a series of episodes when I followed the process as trained, I found myself with a candidate who was so negative in every way that I lost the plot. Instead of sticking to the mandatory questions, I let my emotions rule. I said, well if there is no way you can help me I'll go, and I left the room. Oh dear, I had allowed myself to react as a simulated patient instead of my then role as a standardised patient and thereby undermined the assessment process, leaving the assessors worrying about legal challenge.

A further confusion arises from adoption of the term *human factors*. In the medical world this refers to *'anything that affects a person's performance'* such as personal dexterity or any of the items on the long lists associated with *direct, potential or managing factors*. The Human Factors Model is essential for analysis of team behaviour and particularly apposite in hospital, with its coverage of how people interact with machinery.

The problem has been further compounded recently because 'live' simulators are now used in a cross-over manner in the high-tech world as hybrids with plastic body parts, as accident patients with moulage (theatrical make-up wounds), or as relatives and team colleagues. This adds to the existing confusion because we do, with similar approach and training, simulate doctors to practise performance and appraisal interviews. Add to that the political dialogue around the use of simulation technology that has forced person-to-person simulators (that's another label) to fight for proper recognition in this verbal jungle.

Irrespective of what is going on in the wider world it is necessary to resolve this problem. So, henceforth, in common with others, I use the initials **SP** to stand for simulated patients in medical training and assessment on the understanding that SPs will be real people and furthermore that SPs may also appear as doctors, nurses, health workers, relatives or work colleagues for similar learning purposes. SP

has the virtue that it can be used universally to include standardised or even sample patients. In the USA 'standardised patient' is often used synonymously with 'simulated patient' but it's now more common to regard a standardised patient as one who has been trained to give a highly-specified and consistent performance, as required for high-stake assessment.

The letters SP will refer throughout this text to a person who presents as other than themselves, predominantly as a patient, but on occasions as a doctor, nurse, relative or other, for the purposes of training and assessment of those involved in health care.

Actors or Simulators?

It is common practice to book simulators from actor's agencies. Agencies that have an awareness of health work requirements, for example, suitable cases for a research trial. Almost all simulators work part-time. Institutions requiring simulators either irregularly, or for predictable events spaced throughout the year, therefore need a booking agency. Furthermore, there is a long history of actors being invited and paid to engage in medical training, assessment and research. Nowadays it is not uncommon for student actors to be welcome participants in nurse training; they are keen and they are free! As a result those involved in SP events have frequently been referred to as actors whether they are card carrying members of Equity or not. In my view this poses problems:

- Introducing the term 'actors' into the learning situation may cause unnecessary stress for learners sensitive to being observed by colleagues and can lead others to act in a manner contrary to the way they normally behave. In the context of professional training it is vital that learning is concerned with workplace reality and thus related to normal behaviour. *Using the term 'simulated patient' or SP avoids this problem.*

- SPs may be recruited from people trained in acting or drama schools but that is not to assume that simulating is the equivalent of acting. Though the vocabulary of acting out, role play or performing is inescapable, *the language of acting can divert us from considering what is unique and special about simulating.* Understanding what we are there for is something we need to know, whatever background we come from. Acting a scripted or improvised role in the theatre involves repetition, whereas interacting as a patient is always ephemeral, never repetitive. And it goes without saying that people from a wide range of backgrounds can provide life insights essential for authentic patient presentations.

- Dramatising a patient case is taboo. SPs are required to represent the patient. Insofar as it is possible, SPs are asked to 'be' the patient.

The tension between acting out and representing the patient, doctor, nurse, relative's 'voice' helps us to distinguish between simulating and acting.

To be an SP you need to be able to act out and play a role but simulating is not concerned with acting or role playing in the wider theatrical sense. An actor will take on a role, usually scripted, to <u>become</u> another <u>character</u>, usually in order to <u>project</u> in a <u>predictable</u> way to an audience, for the purpose of entertainment and enjoyment. SPs need to <u>be</u> another person in order to <u>respond</u> to others <u>uniquely and unpredictably</u> as a patient and to represent the '<u>patient voice</u>' in learning and assessment <u>partnerships</u>. To that end SPs are a resource. It is heartening that the formulation of regional simulating policies appear to be avoiding the term 'actor'.

'Being' an SP can have consequences. As Linda with a history of depression I go to the doctor for a vitamin prescription – a friend told me they would help. If I get the prescription I leave, but most doctors don't leave it at that, they delve into my history. On one occasion I did this role for a Simulated Patient Surgery, seeing eight doctors one after the other. All delved. I felt more and more depressed and even found myself crying as I drove home. SP – R G-E

Simulation is a learning resource with its own distinctive methodology

Pioneer **Dr Howard Barrows** First used simulated patients in 1983	Google the History	Pioneer **Dr Paula Stillman** First used simulated patients in 1970

Simulating requires the ability to 'be' rather than to act – 'until the character starts speaking through you you're just someone putting on a voice'.

Anthony Head, actor
Observer Supplement. March 2010

During a 4th Year OSCE I was in bed simulating a seriously ill patient with advanced respiratory problems. The candidate's task was to explain that an arterial blood sample was needed to measure blood gases. This he did. As the bell rang to move to the next station, he whispered in my ear, 'Are you a real patient?' SP - EBW

Simulation for expertise development of health practitioners

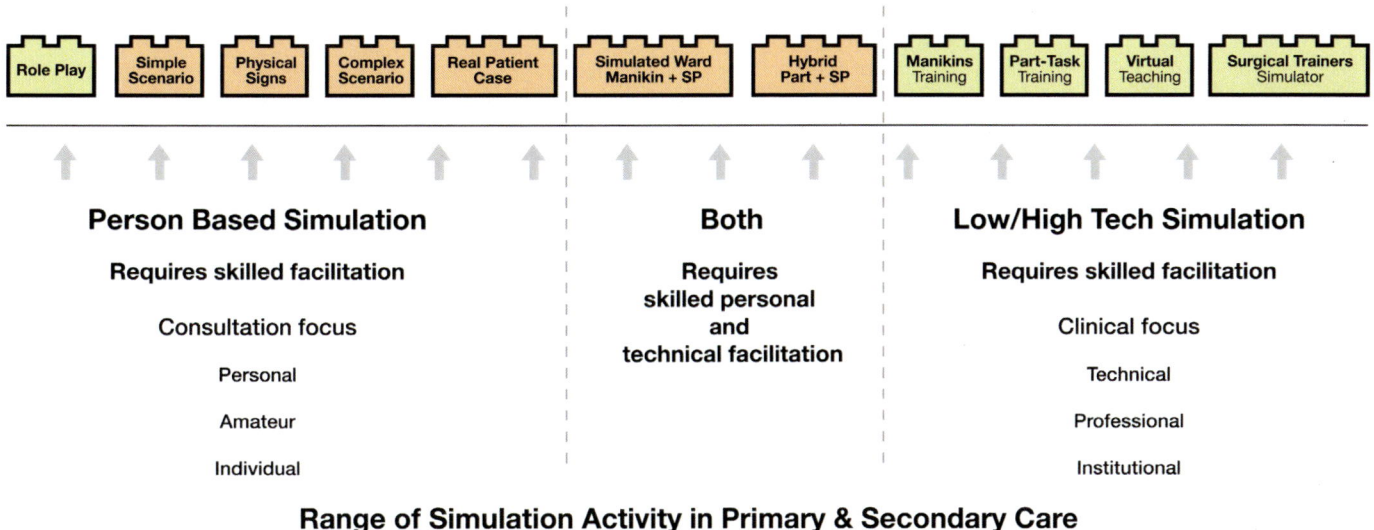

Role Play	Simple Scenario	Physical Signs	Complex Scenario	Real Patient Case	Simulated Ward Manikin + SP	Hybrid Part + SP	Manikins Training	Part-Task Training	Virtual Teaching	Surgical Trainers Simulator

Person Based Simulation

Requires skilled facilitation

Consultation focus

Personal

Amateur

Individual

Both

Requires skilled personal and technical facilitation

Low/High Tech Simulation

Requires skilled facilitation

Clinical focus

Technical

Professional

Institutional

Range of Simulation Activity in Primary & Secondary Care

There is an ever increasing range of learning resources used in medical training. The most recent I've seen is of an avatar representing a pregnant woman designed to illustrate, on screen, what may happen during the birthing process. Dentists use phantom, i.e. plastic heads, to become familiar with handling a head and moving the jaw. Perhaps less exciting and more conventional, the techniques used by SPs are limited to what can happen during person-to-person interactions. The above list of training techniques shows SP activity sandwiched between role play at one end and high-tech processes at the other. Neither role play nor manikins require an SP. The diagram further indicates that SPs require facilitation, usually with a consultation rather than clinical focus and however professionally conducted, are individually responsible practitioners. To date, most SPs work in medical schools and primary or community care.

Simulated wards with manikins provide an example of cross-over with high-tech simulation, in that SPs may be involved as relatives and sometimes as colleagues. They can also appear with moulage wounds for emergency team training.

The boundaries of SP activity

SPs, by definition, play a part in hybrid simulations using add-on plastic body parts to practise procedures, such as catheterisation, together with an obligation to communicate with the patient. Manikins and part-task trainers provide a clear boundary between the work of SPs and the high-tech world. Manikins or part-task trainers, i.e. various dismembered plastic body parts, which are likely to be situated on tables in a laboratory setting for use by clinical instructors, provide a clear-cut boundary – they are inanimate! The boundary marking the human end of the range is more controversial. In the past it has often been customary for SPs to be referred to as role-players – in the sense that you can say taxi drivers play a role within the driving community (my interpretation!). More to the point in boundary marking terms, what is the distinction between role play and simulation?

I was an SP playing the part of a woman who'd been recommended to have surgery. During the consultation the student said, 'When are you planning to have your vasectomy'. Hoots all round. She didn't realise what she'd said so I went on to say, very earnestly, 'Hopefully, very soon'. Even bigger hoots … only then did I say (still in role), 'Do you mean a hysterectomy?'
SP - CO (against the rules but I couldn't resist it)

Role play

Role play is the extempore technique of improvisation. Actors use it to flesh out a character or imagine what might happen so they can interact with each other to build a story. In medicine it can be used to unpack experience with colleagues. An incident with a patient that resulted in a lasting anxiety might be replayed to see how a colleague reacts. Whether or not this elicits greater understanding of your original anxiety or your perception of what the patient might have been feeling, it allows colleagues to share and comment on your problem. Role play has been used ever since GP training became formalised. It featured strongly in Teaching General Practice published in 1981! There are interesting accounts of how to unpack experience by talking to an empty chair and how to alleviate students' reticence in a group with the use of Lego.

Role play can be a powerful, therapeutic technique to share experience, get advice and move on. It does however require very skilled facilitation, willing participants, and of course it has an immediacy that cannot be repeated. Simulations can be repeated. Notwithstanding that, simulators may use some role play techniques to develop a role. Simulations are designed for use in complex learning situations.

More mundanely, simulators get paid. Generating role play for learning requires very particular skills, so role play facilitators may well be paid if they are not staff members.

Role play can be used at any time with a skilled facilitator. It does not require SPs.

The description in Box No 2 illustrates a highly sophisticated, carefully planned form of role play.

A unique example of role play for GP specialty training

Dr Mike Drucquer practices a form of role play that is both challenging and simple, predicated on a patient-centred approach to consulting. He has detailed case scenarios of ten core consulting skills and a further fourteen common consulting problems. He can select any case from this list as appropriate to the GP registrar's learning needs. The cases provide the content. More unique is the manner in which they are used because Dr Drucquer will role play a child, a woman, indeed a patient of any age, gender or cultural background. His registrars know what is required and treat him according to the nature of the scenario, addressing him in an appropriate manner whether as a child, a bereaved mother or whoever.

Dr Drucquer makes no attempt to act. He sits there, is treated in role BUT responds verbally in role according to the scenario. His vast experience with real patients results in authentic replies. Unlike free role play, the interaction, though improvised, is sufficiently authentic for registrar learning. A further unique feature is that the trainer actually experiences how the trainee consults from face to face contact.

The consultation toolkit: a practical method for teaching and learning consultation skills,
Michael Drucquer and Sarah Hutchinson, 2000

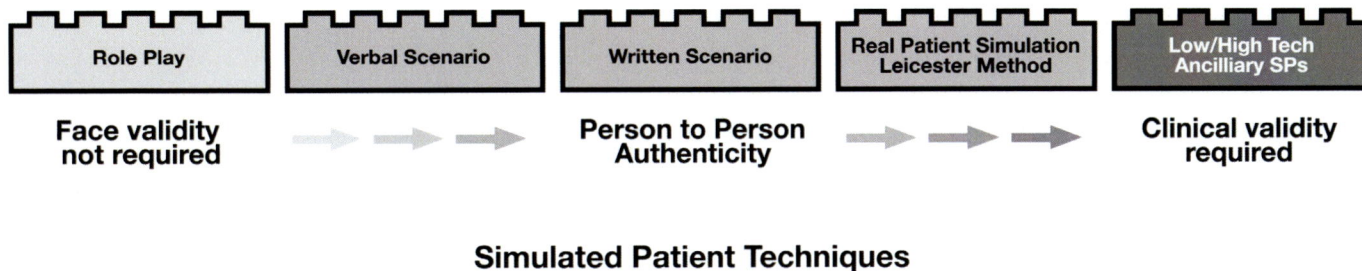

Role Play	Verbal Scenario	Written Scenario	Real Patient Simulation Leicester Method	Low/High Tech Ancilliary SPs

Face validity not required → → → **Person to Person Authenticity** → → → **Clinical validity required**

Simulated Patient Techniques

SPs simulate those involved in both providing and receiving health care. In order to do this for some designated learning purpose there are three commonly used approaches:

1. The simulator may be given a **verbal scenario** of a complexity ranging from a brief summary of <u>who</u> you are, <u>what</u> symptoms you have and <u>why</u> you are here, suitable for a session with receptionists, to one with consultants and senior nurses concerned with cancer patients. Cancer Network promotes a highly articulated course with obligatory training using verbal scenarios concerned with sensitive high-level practitioner issues.

2. **Written scenarios** are by far the most common. Scenarios are used to present a clinical case or situational background for medics, nurses, dentists and other health care students to become familiar with the intricacies of interviewing skills and thereafter to practise them in a variety of professional situations including assessments.

Written scenarios may be as short as two paragraphs; or they may be several pages long, as in the case of a chronic elderly patient with multiple problems of some social and clinical complexity. Scenarios can be composed for a specific learning purpose or, more frequently, chosen from a bank of scenarios designed for, say history taking or concluding a consultation with mutual agreement. Writing scenarios is an art in itself.

It is important that the simulator is able to bond, however loosely with a scenario. Age and gender need to be sufficiently authentic. On receipt of a scenario simulators have to personalise it and ensure that they can portray or recount the symptoms credibly. A scenario is not a script, as the simulator has to respond uniquely to the person consulting.

Written scenarios are similarly used to enable

SPs to become doctors, nurses, relatives and workplace colleagues. SPs become doctors, for example, so that real doctors can practise appraisal or sensitive performance related interviews with colleagues, free of real professional consequences. Over time different SPs may present the same scenario, until, as in my case, age undermines authenticity.

3. More authentic than written scenarios are those SP cases derived from consultations with real patients who've formally consented to being filmed. This approach is less often used because of the time and cost involved. It is worth underlining the fact that developing case material in this way is the nearest SPs come to being able to represent a real patient case.

Agreement has to be negotiated with a GP prepared go through the consent procedure and film a sample surgery. The recording is then scrutinised to select a case which suits a member of the simulating team. The SP then studies the patient in great depth; body language, tone of voice and verbal interchange. Often transcribed verbatim this text becomes the equivalent of a scenario. The doctor and the SP then meet so the SP can question clinical history and current presentation, plus whatever the doctor knows of the social background. The doctor will then consult with the SP to rehearse the case and help with any corrections or omissions. Finally, the doctor will write a condensed set of case notes. These **real patient roles** – still known locally as Leicester Method roles, are usually unique to the originating SP and are rarely transferred to other SPs. Confidentiality is protected throughout and any similarity of name with the original patient is avoided.

Lesser used techniques with SPs include:

* SPs can be taught to replicate a variety of acute cases where recognition of the physical conditions is critical. These may be from primary care, e.g. a frozen shoulder or an

emergency hospital situation such as post-stroke behaviour. These are referred to as physical signs simulations.

- Hybrid simulations require SPs to strap on plastic part-task trainers. For example, women can strap on a birth canal for trainees to practise birthing techniques with the advantage of real patient responses. Similarly, men can strap on a plastic penis for trainee physicians and nurses to practise catheter insertion.

- SPs can also be involved in an important, but more passively emotional way, in complex situations where the learning purpose is 95% clinical. This is the case with the simulated ward with a manikin, where SPs play a minor role as relatives or colleagues. In a similar vein, the day course concerned with organ donation, which follows the pathway of a critically injured patient from delivery by paramedics through to the identification of brain death, requires the presence of relatives. This course is concerned with creating an awareness of the overall procedure for those who may, in their normal working role, only be responsible for a discrete aspect of the pathway progression or be unaware of the sequential decisions required for organ donation, i.e. the clinical pathway is the dominant learning point. As relatives, the presence of SPs is important throughout. Though they must respond as appropriate, their role is more passive than usual because they are primarily there so all concerned can practise involving them appropriately.

The circumstances supporting the two main branches of SP activity are organisationally and economically different. Those involved in high-tech simulation are usually full-time practitioners in stable institutional settings where funding is more secure. SPs are part-timers who work sporadically in a variety of off-site venues. What's more, funding for SPs is limited and vulnerable to allocation changes.

In our region SPs are the roughnecks of the simulation world; a marginal simulation 'modality'.

SPs are mainly concerned with interpersonal skills; whereas, high-tech simulation is mainly concerned with clinical training.

The task of facilitators

At a communications skills workshop it turned out that the participants were not the usual GP trainees but a group of consultants and senior managers. Whilst there is often a reluctance to be the first 'consultor', in this instance it took over half an hour before anyone could be coaxed into the 'hot seat' SP - MS

What distinguishes the work of facilitators? Lectures or demonstrations can engage learners actively or passively in what may be regarded as impersonally large groups. While good lecturers may enliven the process and strongly invite learning, it is still possible to fall asleep, as some of my old notebooks show. Such approaches are necessary for intellectual, didactic learning; learning about **what** to do or think. Whereas, simulation of all kinds is about behaviour, about application; learning **how** to achieve appropriate outcomes. Sometimes, it involves a combination of the interpersonal with the clinical and at others the purely clinical. The task of trainers or instructors is similar, to show people what to do and often to supervise them doing it.

Concerning *'...the facilitation of self-directed learning, that is, with assisting adults to free themselves from externally imposed direction in their learning and with encouraging them to become proactive, initiating individuals in reshaping their personal, work, political, and recreational lives.'*

Understanding and Facilitating Adult Learning, Stephen Brookfield, 1986

With facilitation we move into the field of experience and increasingly into respecting individuals and groups (usually small) as self-learners. Learning for medicine, nursing and other health specialties is predicated on a student pathway to self-learning professionalism; perhaps too exclusively, as will be seen later. To that end facilitation is about enabling learning, the opposite of telling people what to do, and this by facilitating active situations in which students and practitioners can learn according to their current skill level and perception. Facilitators exercise a certain kind of leadership by rarely taking the lead overtly. SPs provide the resource with which the facilitator can manage the interplay of a learning focus, let us say *summarising a case history*, in conjunction with group members and their individual levels of receptivity. The same SP resource may be used for a different focus with more advanced groups, let us say to practise the *negotiation required for mutually agreed treatment*.

Clinicians may have to switch from the training mode essential for inducting trainees into hospital practice, from modelling ward behaviour as experienced nurses or from tutoring GP trainees in primary care, to the more complex approaches required for group learning. SP facilitators may also come from non-clinical backgrounds. From whatever background, facilitators have to juggle a chosen learning focus, individual responses, and sometimes whether or not to follow unplanned learning strands that emerge from interaction with the SP.

Skilled facilitation requires clinicians' willingness to engage with some of the notions that underpin learning activities so they can understand how best to organise learning and then have the language to understand what might be happening during a session. Just as SPs have to become sensitive to aspects of the health world, so facilitators have to become practiced in the arena of a parallel world; the world of learning.
Tucked away on library shelves and learned journals there is ample information concerning the requirements of group facilitation. Unfortunately, it is not always reliably communicated to each new generation of facilitators. I will attempt to do this with specific attention to SP-facilitator expertise.

It is the facilitator's job to juxtapose management of group participation with the declared learning purpose and to maximise individual learning from SP interventions.

I was given a role to test the ability of students to deal with interruptions. The scenario was simple but involved my mobile phone going off. After two minutes my phone rang as planned. I apologised in role and began a simulated reply lasting 30 seconds. The scenario continued for a couple of minutes before my phone rang a second time. At which point the facilitator called 'time out' and asked me to switch off my phone. I was mortified! I couldn't believe that someone could lead a teaching session without knowing the subject matter. SP - EK

Expertise development – the process

The expertise vocabulary in common use derives from the brothers Dreyfus; it follows a progression from novice to advanced beginner to competent to proficient and finally expert. These words reverberate across most professions. The brothers Dreyfus started their enquiries with airline pilots and notable chess players. We now regularly use their language across the various medical specialties and I propose to adopt it to consider the growing expertise of both SPs and facilitators, but in a *tentative fashion*. At the moment there is so little cross-group evidence regarding the work of SPs, or for that matter situations where advanced skills are required, that any determination of progressive expertise must remain at the level of proposals.

We will come to distinguish between the expertise levels achieved by participants when using SPs and the expertise of SPs themselves.

There is of course an overlap, in that competent and proficient SPs will be able to recognise the expertise levels of those with whom they are interacting by acknowledging such qualities, in patient language, when giving feedback.

It is important to note that the work of SPs is by definition complex and the results unpredictable, i.e. emergent; always accepting that the results of bad practice will be more predictable! In any interaction between a patient, individual learners, group observers and the learning task – the customary group learning situation – the outcomes inevitably emerge uniquely. And that's, to use medical argot, contra-indicated in a context where medics and health workers train to achieve greater clinical predictability.

Skilled SPs will not only be capable of representing patients authentically but be able to hold an overview of what is happening in the learning situation. Such an overview will be a sign of higher level expertise.

Interpersonal skills – the content

Whether in the field of business, teaching, entertainment or other fields where person-to-person skills are important, there will always be a number of naturally talented people. In my previous life I estimated that about 15-20% of teachers were naturals in the classroom; they didn't need help with that particular skill. However, SPs' work involves enabling health professionals to interact with patients effectively on different levels: emotional, linguistic, informative or physical. It is therefore necessary to be aware of the language, meaning and application of those interpersonal skills that are most applicable to medical, nursing and health work.

Interpersonal skills provide the learning content for most SP work. Therein lurks a little problem. Patients do not customarily use the somewhat analytical language of interpersonal skills – the distinction between skills and skilled behaviours, for example. Furthermore, it is the job of the SP to 'be' an authentic patient and represent the patient 'voice'. Indeed, when starting out, it is important that new simulators don't clutter their minds with anything other than being the patient. *In role, it is a given that SPs should only respond and give feedback in patient language.* As a consequence, skilled SPs have to keep the analytical language in the back of their minds and constantly find feedback language that avoids technical labelling. For instance, 'summarising' becomes, 'I found it useful when you listed what we talked about because it helped me wonder whether I'd missed telling you something'.

Awareness of interpersonal skill language and sensitivity about its use in practice is an essential attribute of a skilled SP

Having clarified some of the features involved in medical simulating we can now consider a basic starting kit – what needs to be understood as background and what capabilities are required by SPs and those who facilitate learning with them.

Chapter Three
Beginners & Beginnings

If we are to illustrate how the skill of facilitators and SPs might develop over time, there has to be a beginning. Although the necessary practices of both roles are well known, the manner in which beginners are inducted varies from locality to locality – sometimes even according to last-minute pressures. It's not unknown for admin staff to be persuaded to join an SP team and be asked to absorb a scenario by … this afternoon!

Training for beginner SPs can vary from an elaborate recruitment process, followed by several days training, video tapes and advice from well-versed SP team members, to a brief chat and a hand-out. Facilitators likewise may be required to attend a training course on group work theory, or at least be required to sit in with a mentor, rather than take charge of a group with only clinical practice and memories of their own training to guide them – it's happened!

Practice varies from country to country and between localities within each country, so what follows is couched in semi-fictional terms.

The task of an SP is to present as an authentic patient. As a beginner, it is difficult to think of anything other than the character and clinical conditions of the 'someone else' you represent. As confidence grows it will become clear that you are part of a collaborative process – as an educational resource – in company with group participants, a facilitator and a chosen learning purpose.

It is the task of the facilitator to manage the group and its interactions in order to meet the professional learning purpose. Whereas SPs are reactive, the facilitator has to be proactive and reactive and as such bears most responsibility.

The Four Factor Process

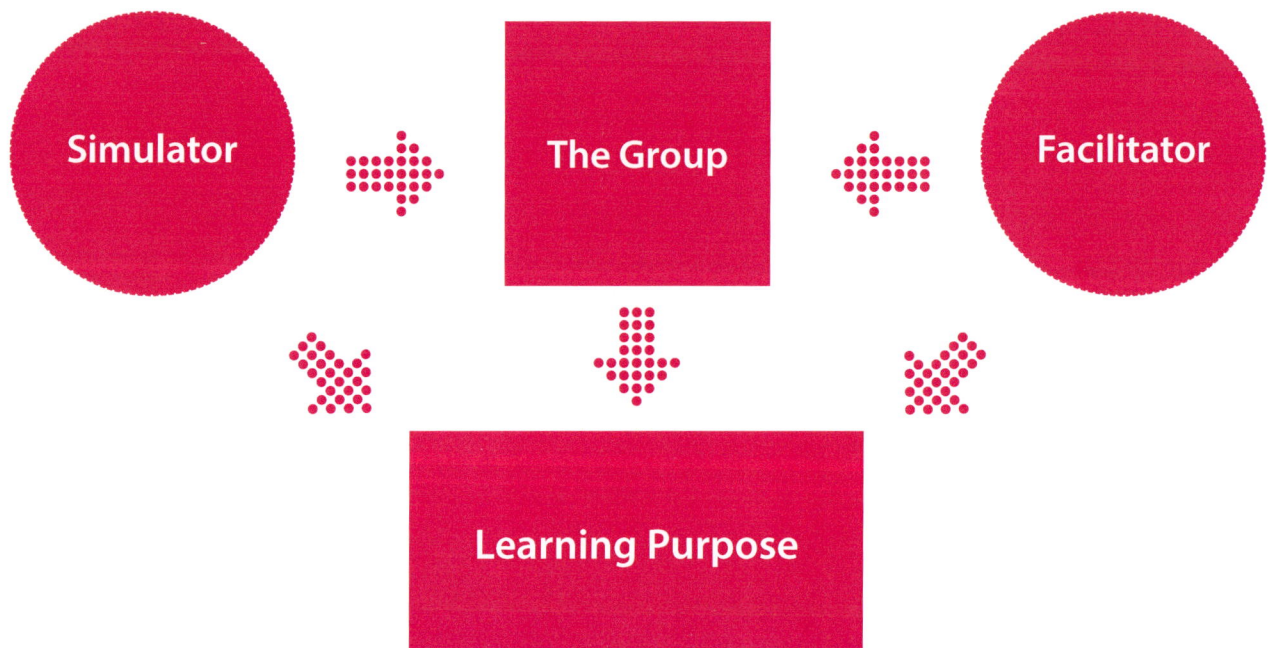

Simulator → **The Group** → **Facilitator**

The Group ↓

Learning Purpose

Beginner Simulator

Best practice for any beginner is to keep things simple. Four decisions govern the following semi-fictional description of a novice becoming an SP. They assume necessary conditions for any locality:

1. A new group of medical students asked to take a patient's history will provide the chosen context, on the basis that such a group will reflect sufficient common practice.

2. A novice simulator will be chosen in order to emphasise lack of prior knowledge about simulation or medical education. In this case the novice simulator is Mrs D, a fictional character. Mrs D is the landlady in Alan Bennett's story, The Greening of Mrs Donaldson, whose student lodger mentions that the medical school is looking for patient simulators. Recruitment procedures have been completed.

3. The approach will be a combination of rudimentary good practice and my own experience.

4. The patient case has been selected from the medical school's case bank in order to avoid a big difference in age and sex between Mrs D and the SP role.

Basic SP Skills

Universal Principles
Understanding the application of equal opportunities
Observing confidentiality

Patient Case
Learning the role
Checking clinical behaviour
Personalising the role

Learning Purpose
Checking group learning level and purpose

In action
Responding in role – consistently
Starting, stopping, winding back
Being examined or providing a findings card
Giving positive, level-appropriate feedback in role

Last week Dr Richard Markham introduced himself to Mrs D as Dr RM, a medical educator and a group facilitator. He explained the general expectations and asked Mrs D to return for a briefing before the group's next session, having read the scenario, worked on a personal and family background and made a clinical timeline of previous medical history. He checked that the presenting symptoms were sufficiently understood to answer a doctor's questions with accuracy.

SP Role Information

Name   Edith Somers

Age   62

CHARACTER

Mrs Somers rarely visits her doctor. She has an open personality and is easy to get on with – she's chatty. She leads an active life and has recently joined a gym as a consequence of which she has become aware of her blood pressure and cholesterol readings. She dresses informally but in accordance with current fashion. She presents as confident which is not surprising as she retired as a teacher two years ago.

SOCIAL HISTORY

Mrs Somers left her husband ten years ago in an amicable divorce. She now lives with her sister. Her daughter who lives nearby relies on her to look after her two primary-school-age grandchildren, including taking them to the doctor. She is an avid reader and a good cook. Once a week she works at the hospice charity book shop.

MEDICAL HISTORY

32 y ago: normal delivery – daughter

8 y ago: fall in school – chest pain – indigestion?

3 y ago: sprained wrist

No regular medicine   Non-smoker   Occasional wine-drinker

REASON FOR ATTENDANCE

Yesterday felt dizzy and fell to the floor in the kitchen.

INFORMATION TO SUPPORT SYMPTOMS

The dizzy feeling is like feeling the room move and as if you might fall – the room seems to be spinning. It makes you want to hold onto something and sit down. It seems to happen when you move your neck or bend down. The feeling goes after about 30 seconds. It's only happened a few times over the past two months. You don't want to make a fuss about it but thought it wise to ask what it might be.

CONCERNS AND EXPECTATIONS

If you feel you are being listened to sympathetically you may volunteer that you're concerned it may be due to a blood pressure problem. You are looking for reassurance and will be reluctant to take any medication.

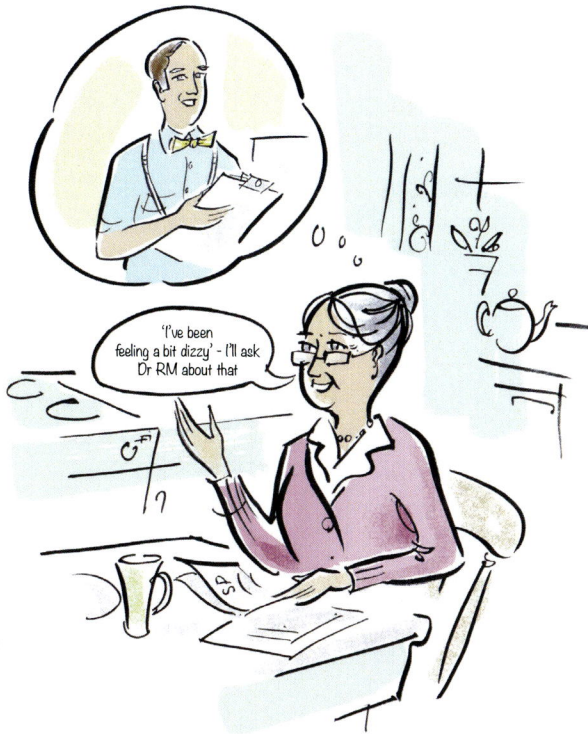

Becoming an SP

Advice from Dr RM

Backstory and clinical timeline

How close do you find Mrs Somers is to yourself? *Oh, very similar in many ways?*
Good, that's why I chose that role. For this first outing feel free to use your own instincts as if they are those of Mrs Somers, if you can't quickly imagine how Mrs Somers might respond [1]. Otherwise bring in the backstory [2] – that's the word we use for the personal and family history. How does she walk and sit? What sort of handbag does she carry? Family members? This kind of thing is up to you! As you introduce aspects of her life not included in the scenario, remember that they then become an unwritten part of the role in the future – that's for you; others would do it to suit their own inclinations.

Symptoms – the clinical expectations

I explained the nature and likely treatment for her dizziness at our last meeting. Year one students are asked to take a history so you won't be offered a diagnosis. You think it might be a blood pressure problem but only disclose this if you think they are really concerned with your welfare. It says you want reassurance. *About what? –Falling?* Use your own feelings about this and the effects it has on your lifestyle. Could it happen in the street or in the supermarket? Has it kept you in?

Basic practice

* Remember how the person consulting greets you
* Use the same or similar opening statement
* If you don't know the answer to a question, just say, 'I don't know'
* Challenge unusual questions: 'Why are you asking that?'
* Consider carefully how you think inner disclosures might be received
* As far as possible remember what is said and watch for non-verbal clues
* Question the meaning of medical terms you don't understand

Feedback

As facilitator, I will ask for your feedback in role – please answer in Mrs Somers's everyday language.

[1] Sometimes novices are given a clinical scenario and asked to present it as themselves with no alternative characteristics.

[2] Referred to later as the process of 'personalisation'.

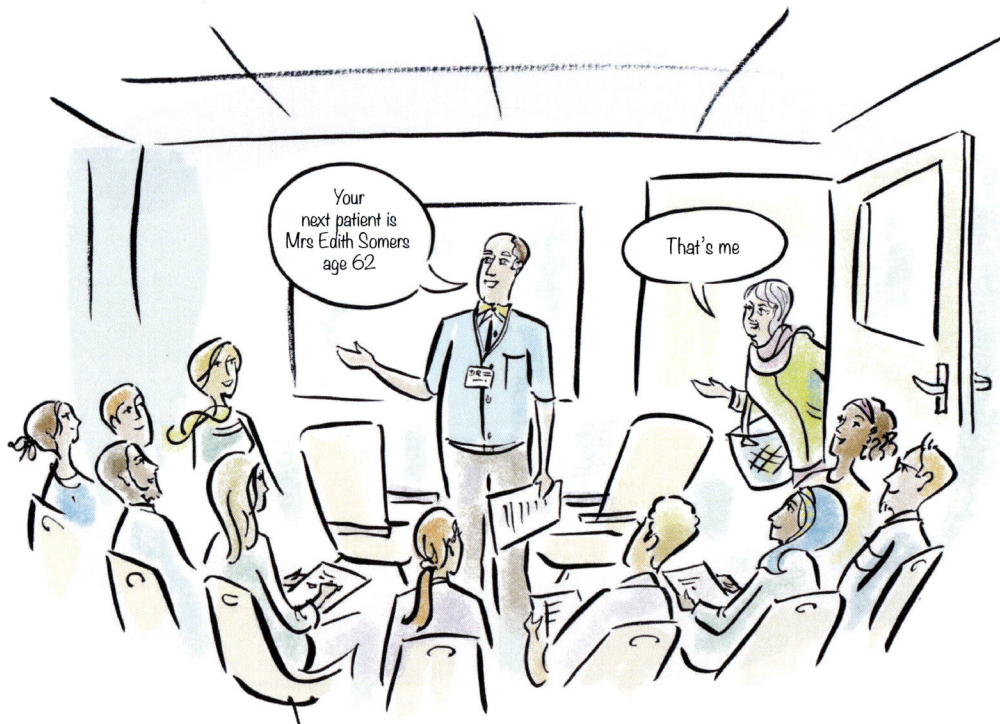

Group learning

Setting up the group

I always arrive before the group so I can organise the room. For example, I make sure the two chairs for the patient and the person consulting are in a clear line from the door. We don't want you climbing over people to get in! On this occasion I suggest you sit by the open door so you can hear what I'm saying to the group. That'll give you background to the session's purpose and plan.

- I'll check the register and identify who is to consult next – there will be an opportunity for three of the group to consult with you. This is why we talk about 'cleansing' – being able to start afresh as if each is a first-time consultation.
- I'll recall last week's session, remind them that we are still concerned with history taking and find out if there are things they would like to try out or explore!

Group processes

- With this novice group I'll need to remind them about such things as 'time-out', and observing and recording what is said and seen for feedback purposes.
- As we are considering history taking we will limit each consultation to about five minutes; plus, in each case with the opportunity to continue and try alternative techniques.
- The patient is called Mrs Edith Somers, aged 62. As this will be a first time consultation, it's up to the person consulting to find out your previous medical history, reasons for attending, etc.

Learning purposes

- As always we have two learning purposes in parallel. There is history taking with its sub-text of finding the patient's ideas, concerns and expectations, together with practising specific interpersonal skills. In this case we are focusing on open and closed questions, use of silence, summary and sensitivity to non-verbal expression.
- Pen and paper out, I want this half of the group to record history taking evidence and the rest to record specific instances of the interpersonal skills.
- OK. Let's call in the patient.

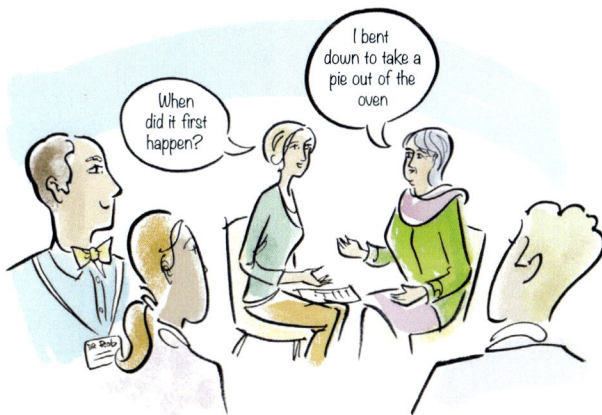

Action - SP in the chair

Commentary - Thoughts of an experienced observer

Greeting

How patients are greeted illustrates the difference between social and professional life. Socially we may greet people casually and with little thought – it's a routine. But if a doctor treats a patient casually – maybe with indifferent eye contact and tone of voice, or without looking up from the computer – there are often consequences. A patient may not disclose intimate detail to such a doctor or adopt an 'I don't want to bother you' approach. This is a point worth labouring because it highlights the value of using SPs to consider the consultation in detail. The task is to react and recall. For example, many doctors often mumble their name, so the SP can play the innocent and say, 'Sorry, Dr ...? – making sure the name is clearly known.

Responding

It is the person consulting whose behaviour is really in the spotlight (if the patient is sufficiently authentic). So, Mrs D as Mrs Somers makes her opening statement and pauses. The Year One medical student uses open and closed questions to explore her medical history, and Mrs Somers responds appropriately. That's fine. But what happens if the person consulting pauses and

their eyes say they are waiting for her to continue telling the story? What does she say? How long is the silence kept? It happens. The third student in the chair does pause. How long will Mrs Somers keep the silence? Oh, she plays safe and says, *'What else do you want to know?'* Only the SP knows what to do in a silence, based on interpretation of the scenario and the patient's backstory.

Time out

Dr RM calls 'time out' at various points in the sequence of consultations. Each time, Mrs Somers goes quiet and looks down – no eye contact. She assumes she's not there until the prompt to continue. On one occasion, she's asked to return to a previous point in the consultation. Later she's asked to return to the chair outside the door. Is she erasing what's just happened, i.e. cleansing? Maybe hearing what Dr RM has been discussing about what to do next will have helped to change the scene. Yes, as she's called in she uses her opening statement and a different interview unrolls.

Cleansing

Nothing to do with washing hands, this concerns the need to free your mind from anything that has happened in the previous episode. Think of yourself as a resource, such as a projector which you can switch on and off. As one consultation follows another you need to start afresh, as if you have never talked to anyone before about your dizziness.

Cleansing is a skill. In one half of your mind you may remember what happened previously, but you put it aside for the moment.

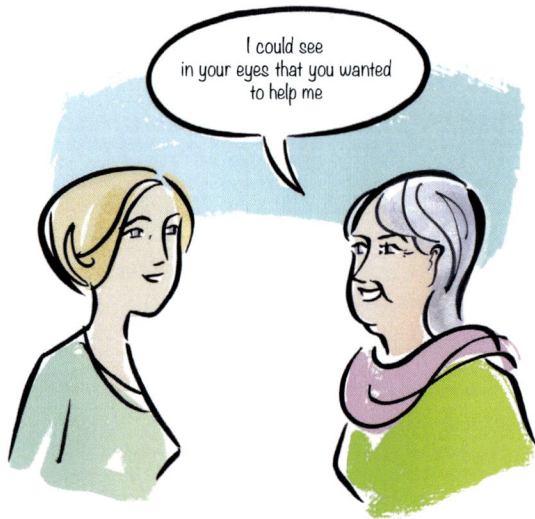

I could see in your eyes that you wanted to help me

Giving feedback

Thoughts of an experienced observer – continued

Feedback routines

The group facilitator, Dr RM in this case, followed the routine agreed with the group at the beginning. He first asked the consultor what she did well. Next he asked what the observers saw and heard and then returned to ask the consultor what she might have done differently – a routine known as Pendleton's rules (from *The Consultation: An Approach to Learning and Teaching* by Pendleton et al). Only then was Mrs Somers asked. Dr RM helped with specific questions to elaborate on points made by the observers, thereby avoiding the requirement for her to conjure up her own feedback. Feedback routines vary according to the learning tasks.

Recalling what happened

There was feedback after each short consultation so what happened was fresh in Mrs Somers's mind. This will not always be the case, particularly with long consultations. Concentrating on 'being' the patient sometimes makes recalling what happened difficult, but there are little verbal tricks to get round this.

Using lay, non-technical language

The rule is, never use technical language for in-role feedback. Easily said, but sometimes difficult to achieve, e.g. 'You gave me time to think' is common language for the technical phrase, 'use of silence'. Though rare, you may be called upon to play someone who is genuinely knowledgeable or who may come armed with information from the internet, in which case you may relish breaking the rule to use technical language of a mystifying kind.

Feedback in role

One powerful attribute of learning with SPs is the benefit of receiving feedback in the 'patient voice'. To that end, Mrs Somers did concentrate on giving feedback as the patient, which is good for a first experience. Only once did Dr RM have to protect her from giving out-of-role feedback – she would need to be much more aware of the technical language used in professional training to be at risk of doing this.

Feedback rules

- Check if feedback required in or out of role or both
- Focus on observed behaviour, not the person
- Focus on what is seen and felt (immediacy)
- Focus on description rather than judgement (no value judgements)
- Focus on specific behaviours in the context they occur

Giving constructive feedback is a complex skill that grows with experience. For this first attempt, limit yourself to uncomplicated statements of feeling and only then if they are supportive, e.g. very neutrally, I was able to say all I needed to, or more positively, it was easy talking with you. Beware of making value judgements outside the role of patient, e.g. I thought you took a good history of my case. As a patient you would know nothing about medical history taking! Stick to making observations on what happened

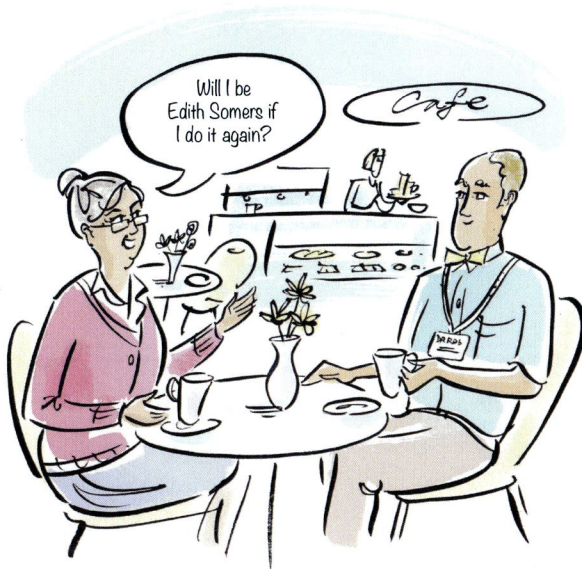

Debrief with Dr RM

How was it for you?

Mrs D: *Well, as I sat there outside the room, my head was in turmoil. When the person consulting said, 'Come in Mrs Somers', I just smiled, went in and sat down. Luckily, I remembered to say, 'I've been having these dizzy spells', and then waited, like you said. After that I just answered the questions and began to relax and look around. They are young, aren't they?*

What I saw you doing

Dr RM: *Whatever was going on in your mind, you appeared to be very natural and composed to me so you came over as a real patient. And you did as you were told by responding not leading, so there were no gaffs. Although you know the dizziness is not serious, you came over as a worried Edith – just what we wanted.*

Some practical issues

Dr RM: *What do you feel was useful in taking on your role?* **Mrs D:** *Imagining Mrs Somers' backstory did give me confidence. As I sat there, knowing her story, I was surprised how little it was used. There was just the one question about who keeps an eye on me at home.* **Dr RM:** *That one question shows the values of your backstory. It made your SP life real.*

You had three consultations as the same person, were you the same person every time?

Mrs D: *I was the same person every time but different every time, if that makes sense.* **Dr RM:** *Makes perfect sense to me. That's real life and good simulating. The question is, were you consistently the same? Was the story consistent, however it emerged? And while we are on about consistency, never change the clinical details.*

What next?

Dr RM: *Now you've had a go, how do you feel about doing it again?* **Mrs D:** *It's another world isn't it? There I was sitting in a room, surrounded by students, wrapped up in the medical concerns of Edith. There was such a level of concentration; what was happening clearly mattered. It's catching! And I get a little cheque! Can I have another go?* **Dr RM:** *You're welcome. Can you come next Wednesday?*

Consistency

Consistency applies to the content of the case, i.e. do not go outside the boundaries of the scenario, as you have personalised it. Unless you are obliged to answer a question to which you have to provide an answer not covered in the scenario, do it in role – as you would imagine Edith would reply. Your response must henceforth become part of the scenario in order to maintain consistency.

Do not confuse content consistency with the manner of response, as this will vary according to who you are talking with.

Afterthought

We learn from Erving Goffman (*The Presentation of Self in Everyday Life* – 1959) that we act so that we will, intentionally or not, express ourselves in such a way that others will be impressed. With that in mind, it is important for SPs to be aware of how they normally present – check with others. With that awareness we can adapt to present as others.

For this first experience Mrs D was asked to **use** her own life experience to fill out the character of Edith Somers but, perhaps it wasn't emphasised that we must never be **ourselves** as SPs; that's the 'self' we actually take to the doctor. It has been known for a simulator to slip in a question about a personal ailment and thus ignore the 'non-contamination by self' rule – a red card situation.

New Facilitator

Keeping things simple for a new facilitator has one drawback. While SPs may be said to come with prior life experience, maybe even with relevant teaching or drama skills, and often with experience as a real patient, they are unlikely to know much about medical education. Given that most facilitators will be doctors, nurses or health workers from various backgrounds, potential facilitators will inevitably have strong recollections from their own education and training. Unlike the SPs, they may even have ideas about what and how their future colleagues should learn. They may have facilitated groups using other learning techniques, for example the digital storytelling of patient experiences pioneered by *Patient Voices*.

Bearing in mind the need to think of facilitation from a fresh point of view, in this fictional scenario I have made four decisions in order to approach the task with as clean a sheet as possible.

1. The learning context will be in the nature of a 'one off', unlikely to be repeated or even experienced by most medical educators. It concerns a group of twelve experienced nurses who have been involved in a postgraduate course to become nurse prescribers. The end-of-course assessment will involve consultations with simulated patients. Most, maybe all the nurses, will have no previous experience with SPs. In order to lessen anxiety, they have been offered a familiarisation session.

2. Cheryl, a nurse educator from an introductory nurse training scheme has volunteered to facilitate a half group of six nurses. Elaine the course director, who will manage the other half group, has promised to mentor her.

3. The familiarisation case has been constructed to enable candidates absorb the pattern of likely assessment criteria during the SP consultation.

4. Both SPs booked for the session are experienced simulators.

Basic Facilitator Skills

Temperament
Calm & Measured
Non-directive

Universal Principles
Understands application of equal-ops in groups
Constantly works towards self and group determined learning

Clear processes
Seating – Use of SP – Group tasks - Observation – Making mistakes – Trying new approaches – Feedback rules

In action
Keeping time – Use of challenge – Switching control – learning check

---

Elaine explains the session's purpose to Cheryl

'I know you've been to this centre before and seen the rooms. There's the bigger one for the whole-group introduction and a smaller break-out room. I suggest you take the smaller room, it's more intimate and you only need to arrange the chairs in the way you prefer. These are very experienced nurses who've worked in a variety of situations but most are attached to GP practices. Surprisingly, given their clinical expertise, they're very nervous about the assessment and more so about consulting with an SP – and even more so about consulting in front of their colleagues. As you well know, they normally consult alone. In the foreground of this session is the need to help them feel comfortable consulting with an SP. It's also an opportunity to show how they'll be observed. Their history taking and prescribing will form the background of the assessment. I've written the following scenario to illustrate the level of challenge they'll face during the assessment:'

SP Role Information

Patient   Lawrence West

Age   46

SOCIAL BACKGROUND

Married – Children aged 14, 16 & 19 – Self-employed painter and decorator

MEDICAL BACKGROUND

7 years ago: Well man check NAD
3 years ago: Fell off ladder, fractured arm
1 year ago: Foreign travel injections

Occasional smoker   social drinker

REASONS FOR PRESENT APPOINTMENT

You've had a cough for 5 days or so. It started with a prickliness in the throat, then you felt a bit poorly and think you had a slight temperature. That's gone away but you are now coughing up yellow spit. Your wife has insisted you get it seen to and you can't afford to be off work if it gets worse. Getting work is becoming increasingly stressful. You think that's why you may be getting indigestion.

If asked you will say you have not coughed up blood and not felt breathless. You have not had a chest problem in the past and there is no history of chest problems in your family, as far as you know. You limp slightly on entering the surgery and carry a walking stick. If asked about the limp you tell the doctor that you have recently twisted your ankle (no swelling). To ease the pain you have been taking Ibuprofen – you think about 4 per day.

EXPECTATIONS

You hope the doctor will prescribe something to clear up your cough or tell you what to get from the chemist.

CHARACTER

You are a matter of fact man of action who copes without saying much. You tell it as it is. You think the leg will mend but it's the work stress that's uppermost in your mind.

Lawrence West • Patient Checklist	YES	NO
The nurse asked me to describe my cough.		
The nurse explained that the cough would probably get better on its own and that I should come back if my temperature comes back, my spit goes green or I become breathless.		
I explained why I was using a stick		
I understand I was taking too much Ibuprofen which might be causing my indigestion		
I did not get a prescription for my cough.		

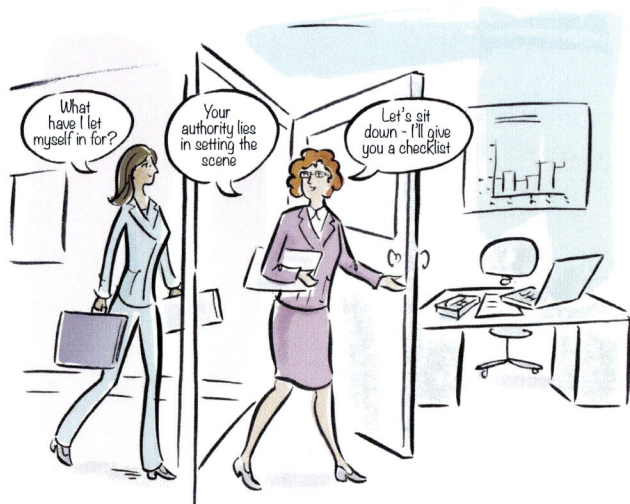

Becoming a Facilitator

More advice from Elaine

Reminders

There are some members of this course you will warm to more than others. Though I'm sure you will be even-handed, you need to know we've had complaints in the past. The assessment is our equal opportunities moment, so please give everyone an equal chance to consult and receive feedback according to the rules. Our group work with these experienced practitioners is underpinned by the notion of self-directed learning. Give them the opportunity to learn by doing, i.e. by putting into practice what they have learnt using the simulated patient. Mistakes, and one hopes there will be some, are there for everyone's learning. You can help them apply 'course learning', as opposed to 'clinical direction'.

Your authority

I'll introduce you but they will be wary of a new face. Your authority will reside in setting the scene and the way you manage their experience with the SP.

Setting the scene

Here's the checklist I use:

- Get there first and set the room up with a clear path from door to chair for the SP.

- Meet the SP, check case details and that SP appreciates nature of group learning. We work with SPs on a one-off basis with colleagues like you who we press-gang into facilitating. To help you, we've written a 'Working with SPs' hand-out.

- Outline session purpose and process – include reassurance about assessment

- Check previous experience with SPs. Explain time-out practices, agree consulting sequence and emphasise ability to try new approaches. Mention feedback from group after each consultation, and that there will be an SP case changeover after the tea break, so everyone will have a face-to-face opportunity.

Feedback for you

We'll debrief afterwards but I suggest you work out some way to get the group's reaction as to the usefulness of the session. This might also be a useful way to conclude and, knowing how worried some are, to provide reassurance by relating what you saw happening as good practice.

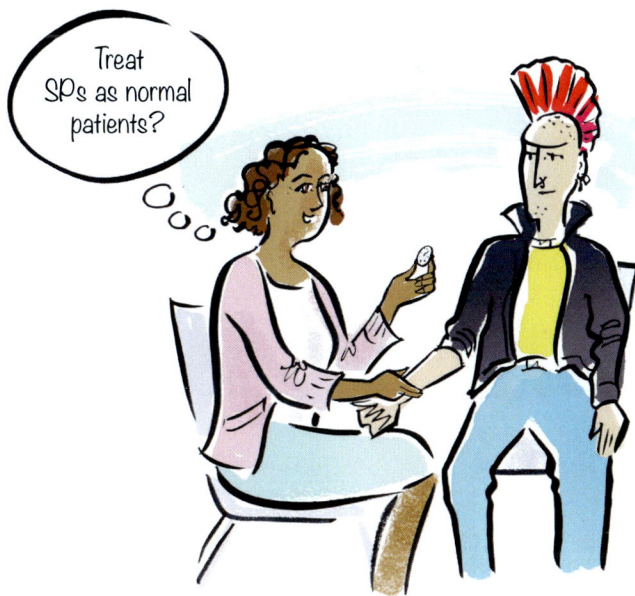

The SP needs to know the learning purpose in order to temper responses to that end.

- You can stop, start and rewind the consultation by using 'time out'. On hearing 'time out' the SP will blank out. You may do this to highlight a learning point or suggest a changed approach. Be aware that the SP will hear everything that's going on and will therefore know, without being told, to start again where the consultation stopped, or rewind to a previous point, or respond to a 'let's try' suggestion. You may wish to ask the SP to leave the chair in order to be called in for a greeting each time the person consulting changes over.

- You will normally explain the feedback procedures at the beginning of the session, with particular attention to the feedback sequence, e.g. consultor first, followed by group observations and finally the SP. A consultation may be stopped after a specified time, say 3 minutes, to see how much information has been obtained and to discuss the presenting problem. If you wish SPs to contribute at this point, please forewarn them so they can feedback appropriately – it may simply be, 'how are you feeling at this point?'

- It is not easy for SPs to give meaningful summary feedback at the end of a session. They have to concentrate so hard they may have forgotten what happened an hour before. But they will almost certainly be able to respond to specific questions from you or the group.

The SP Hand-out

Working with a Simulated Patient (SP) Information for Facilitators

- The SPs we use have experience across a range of healthcare training, most of which involves small group learning, so they instinctively know how to fit your needs.

- They receive a scenario, such as the Lawrence West case, from which they absorb the outline clinical and character details. They then personalise the role by creating a personal history and a family background.

- Facilitators need to introduce themselves and exchange information. You should become familiar with the case, the patient's character and how that will impact on disclosure and treatment decisions. SPs frequently need to check on the clinical aspects of the role so they can answer and behave accordingly. In some cases SPs can be examined. In others, the SP will have examination results on a card. Participants should be informed of the examination protocols when appropriate. We recommend that you ask the SP to give feedback in role.

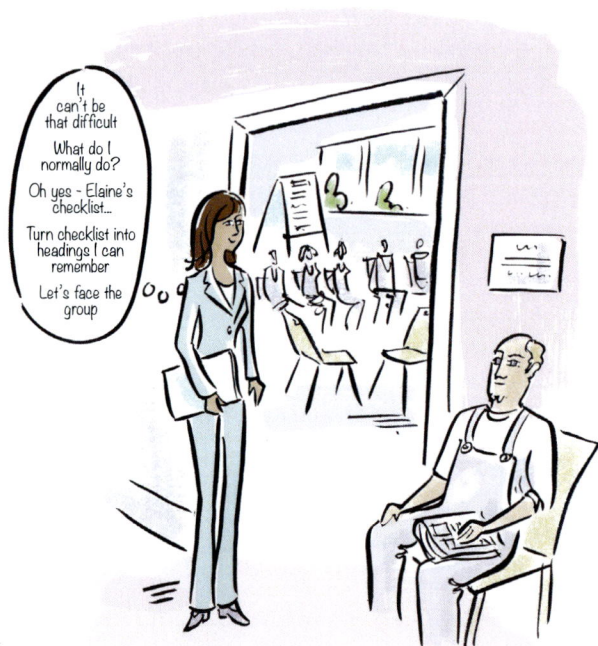

Preparatory Thoughts

Knowns

- I've run learning groups before
- The purpose is to raise confidence
- There will be six experienced nurses aspiring to become nurse prescribers
- Everything revolves around a simulated patient

Unknowns

- How best to work with an SP?
- How nervous experienced nurses respond in a high-stake learning group?
- How to build up confidence as a group activity?

This shines a light on my insecurity so I'll put that aside and concentrate on the 'authority' Elaine talked about. First, I've taught for years AND run learning groups, albeit with inexperienced nurse trainees. Second, all the unknowns will remain unknown until I've had the experience, so I'll organise my learning curve with a to-do list and just get on with it.

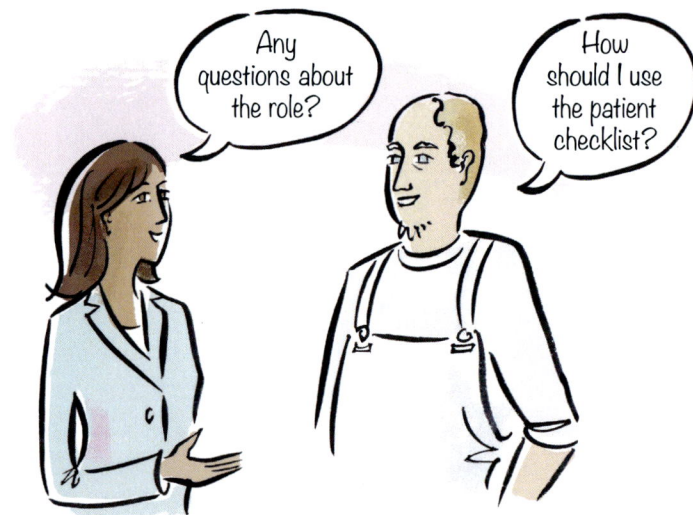

Action

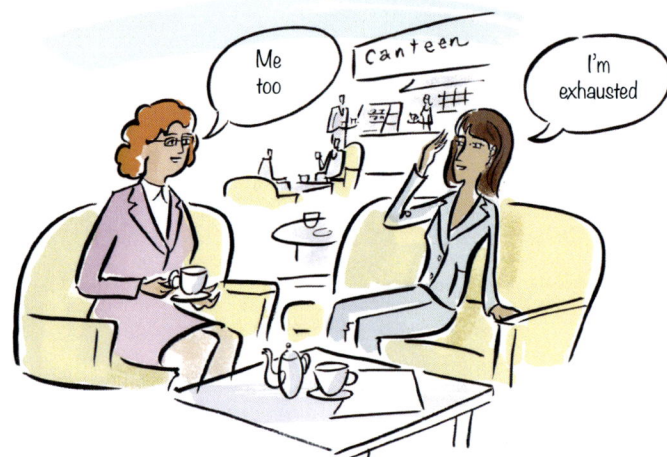

Debrief

Did it happen? Debrief with Elaine

Was the room suitable for group learning?

I arranged the chairs before anyone arrived as you suggested. That meant I could greet them individually as they arrived. Otherwise, it was just a plain room with a flipchart. As for the SP, rather than sit him outside, I arranged for him to sit at the back of the room so he could hear the briefing.

How did you interact with the SP?

We chatted about Lawrence West to start with. He'd done the role before so it was clinically sound and there was no call for an examination. The time-outs worked well and he gave some individually perceptive feedback. At the end he said he enjoyed working with me, which was reassuring.

How did you get on with the group?

I'm not really sure; they were six such different people. They ranged from silent to garrulous and from overly patient centred to consulting on auto-pilot. By keeping good time we managed to follow the procedure I'd outlined and to my surprise actually give colleague feedback on a what-you-hear-what-you-see basis. Mind you I'm used to being fierce about this when my students analyse DVD recordings. Four out of six would have ticked all the checklist boxes and only one gave a prescription – the others were a bit smug about this. Familiarisation wise, knowing what to expect at the assessment went through on the nod.

What about the nature and quality of feedback?

It was all positive but I think this was because they already knew each other's sensitivities. Also perhaps, because the more confident nurses did the initial consultation for each case, and frankly, because of the helpful SP feedback.

Do you think the session achieved its learning purpose?

From what they said, the answer is 'yes', unless they were being polite. At another level I'm not sure what they learnt. From an evidence point of view, they concentrated throughout, they followed the procedures and – maybe this is the most indicative – whatever their reservations, they all treated the SP as they would a real patient.

And what did you get out of it?

I listened to your advice – it had a strategy in-built. Then I thought, what do I normally do? I'm not entirely new to this game. So I turned your checklist into a list of headings I could remember and

followed them, both in setting the scene and more importantly, keeping to time. That's Lesson One for me; Headings – Time – Task. Three nurses had a 10-minute consultation plus feedback, and there was still time, before the tea break, for somebody to have 3 minutes in the chair to try a different approach. I did exactly the same for the next SP case. As for the learning purpose, well that's Lesson Two for me: achieving really good results lies both in setting the scene (there's more than one way to do it!) and in how you react to what's going on – the unpredictable element.

The concentration required is extraordinary.

Chapter Four
Facilitiating Learning in Small Groups with Simulated Patients

Across specialties, health care practitioners are accustomed to learning by means of lectures, practicals, demonstrations, tutorials, assessments and e-learning, all feeding into and reinforced by work-based experience. Recently there's been an increase in simulated work-related learning with manikins and high-tech simulators. Most conventional learning is task orientated, and is presented to passive or semi-passive trainees by means of traditional teacher-tutor methods – university tutors are trained in these methodologies and the educational ideas that validate them. To a large extent clinical specialists have been able to train others by modelling good practice with only a modicum of learner-centred theory. This can also apply to group work using SPs as the resource, i.e. focus on a required behaviour and practise it with an SP.

Group work has a developmental history parallel to customary learning practices. Its development precedes the use of simulators. Group work has been used as a cauldron for changing the behaviour of recidivists. Balint introduced group work for practising GPs to unpack and reflect on their day-to-day practice. Therapeutic groups abound. Significantly, group learning of all kinds is facilitated rather than tutored. Indeed, the term facilitation implies a more indirect approach to learners, which in turn, implies that learners will need to assume more responsibility.

Group work is by nature interactive. Add a simulated patient to the group mixture and it becomes even more active. Because of its closeness to real practice, it translates into experiential learning suitable for development of professional expertise. Of course, group dynamics will be affected by participants' characters and learning styles, their stage of learning, the learning context, the nature of SP cases, facilitator experience, and group numbers – the list can go on. It is the facilitator who unlocks the learning potential door, assisted by more experienced SPs.

So, why learn about learning? Knowing what you are doing becomes essential given the multiple factors in play and the need for rapid decision making. Group work with an SP is an approach that can reveal insights into why and how things might be done differently; it involves group members in collaborative tasks, illuminates the reasoning behind learning behaviours, takes into account workplace demands. It's an educational approach that achieves more than one thing at a time. Michael Eraut puts it rather differently:

> *Unless they [facilitators] can conceptualise the task of learning to theorize they are unlikely to develop the capacity to do so.*
>
> Michael Eraut,
> Developing Professional Knowledge and Competence, 1994

Learning pathways for professional educators follow two parallel routes: first, application, learning what to do and how to achieve it; second, recognition and understanding of what might be going on, having an overview of what you are doing, for which the educational term is metacognition! The two routes converge on issues involved in the group learning dynamic.

MAKING IT HAPPEN

APPLICATION

Application

Knowing HOW to prompt activity that will lead to better understanding and changed levels of expertise is driven by understanding HOW people learn

'KNOWING'

Metacognition

Having enough analytical language to know what you are doing at any one time and having the educational language to plan ahead provides the potential for high expectations

Application

Influential factors in an active learning group

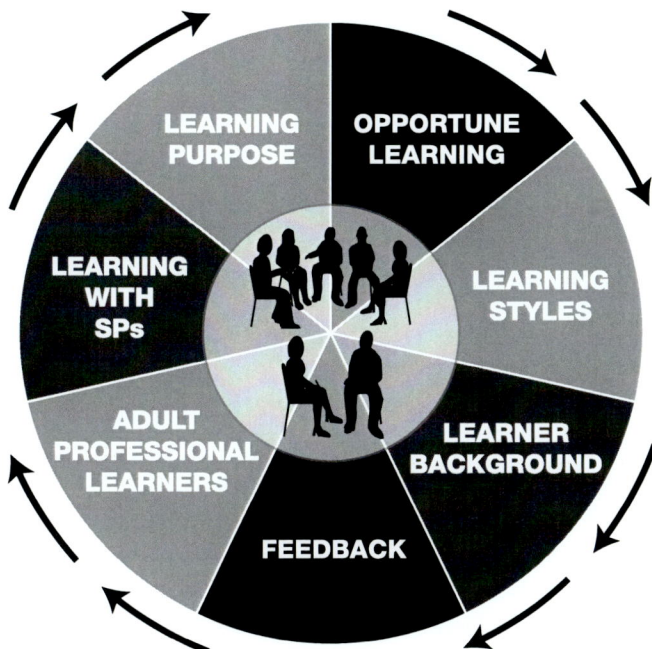

LEARNING PURPOSE · OPPORTUNE LEARNING · LEARNING STYLES · LEARNER BACKGROUND · FEEDBACK · ADULT PROFESSIONAL LEARNERS · LEARNING WITH SPs

Working with Adult Professional Learners

Adult learners come with considerable amounts of prior experience, some of which may be useful and some of which needs to be unlearnt. It is important to assume that adults will learn idiosyncratically. They may need time, not only to digest new ideas but time and opportunity before new ideas are translated into behaviour – sometimes this means never!

- It is useful to challenge the meaning behind individual actions in order to *reinforce* that which is positive, share it, and compare it with the views of others.

- Prior learning may explain why members may say they have learnt nothing, or perhaps, nothing new. But the extension or reaffirmation of previous learning may be equally valuable.

- Adults may have strong predispositions, e.g. cultural or social prejudices, which have to be suppressed or encouraged. Professionals are obliged to regard their patients or clients with 'unqualified positive regard', to quote Carl Rogers's powerful advice. Ensuring this is 'lived out' can be a struggle.

Please note; there is a powerful assumption that all professional learners have a **self-determined learning** agenda; that they are indeed 'adult learners'. Beware: some may be waiting to be 'told'. There should be evidence that 'adult learner status' has been earned.

'To engage in the collaborative exploration and interpretation of individual experience is the most meaningful form of discussion for adults'

Stephen Brookfield,
Understanding and Facilitating Adult Learning, 2001

Responding to Learner Backgrounds

One obvious factor regarding the potential to learn is the level of training currently achieved, from post school to practitioner, juxtaposed with the content of learning appropriate to the particular branch of the health service, i.e. is the learning focus **appropriate?** Add to this the cultural nature of prior learning, if that was in a different country. Differences need to be made explicit in order to avoid misunderstandings. In practice this ranges from issues such as the obligation to provide chaperones to more intangible matters. For example, in UK general practice the deference to patients' wishes can be difficult for doctors brought up in countries where doctors have high, relatively unchallengeable status.

- Awareness of learning levels can be vital to avoid tedious repetition or talking above people's heads during initial learning but this is usually standardised through institutional curricula. Group work with SPs is usually well matched to learning need. Facilitators still need to check understanding at individual levels, to ensure there is personal learning progression.

- It's interesting to be aware that there are four 'learner' contexts in an SP focused group – the consultor – the observers, each with a different learning engagement – the facilitator regarding effectiveness – the SP by adding depth to the person of the patient.

Recognising Learning Styles

Individuals come with learning styles best suited to them. This is most apparent on a one-to-one discussion basis. To an extent group learning enables people to learn at their own pace and in their own style.

It is still useful to recognise levels of **receptivity** which, at a fundamental level, involves three learning domains:

cognitive = thinking
affective = feeling
psychomotor = doing

While some veer along one path or other, for example, intellectuals along the cognitive path, most of us (thankfully) can claim a bit of each level.

Another noticeable learning style distinguishes between those who learn better aurally or visually or, again thankfully for most of us, some of both. Then there is the dependent to independent spectrum between those who prefer to be told and those who want to learn for themselves. There's no doubt which end of that spectrum is necessary for group learning! Most important is what might be called the sociological spectrum, which reflects confidence, expressiveness, collaboration, maybe even altruism.

In a self-learning culture some medics with a strong cognitive aptitude may retain a dependent, less flexible, learning style which they modify in training to gain patient-centred assessment success, but then revert to their natural disposition when the pressure is off!

- The overriding secret of productive group work is to: personalise the role of yourself and the SP; clarify the learning purpose and its scope; model openness and fairness, i.e. set it up so that people with different learning styles can feel free to express themselves collaboratively. Forget any analysis of personal learning styles until there is a noticeable difficulty.

- Awareness of some learning styles (there are more!) can be useful if, for example, a group member becomes exasperated: 'Why are we endlessly discussing this when you know what we ought to do in practice – why not just tell us?' You will recognise the dependent learner and know how to deal with them. Prefacing a response with, 'Well what I would do is …' would, for instance, provide a direct answer while preserving the notion that most health practitioners act individualistically.

Learning with SPs

Most people tend to take learning with SPs for granted after they've had an initial session 'in the chair'. Some continue to find what they see as the artificiality of the so-called patient difficult to cope with. This may well be compounded by the personal exposure required to 'act out' in a group of watching colleagues. Dealing with this at the time is not difficult; protect the member's public self-esteem and maybe negotiate a compromise. For those who cannot adjust there are long-term difficulties because simulation plays a part in important assessment procedures: OSCEs and college membership exams.

- The degree of firm handedness required depends on group size and continuity. A group of four, the minimum advised, can be treated informally. It's different when there are twelve.

- It is advisable to remind members of the necessary processes: 'time out', patient examination protocols, observation for feedback and the possibility to try things out safely. The opportunity to try different personal approaches soon identifies the independent learners!

- With written scenarios there is an opportunity to agree a change in the way the patient presents, e.g. more assertively or less openly. It is acceptable to change the role to suit a particular learning request as long as the changes involve the patient's personality and not the medical aspects.

- *N.B. It was common in the past for facilitators to invite a group member to sit in the 'hot seat'. Given the anxiety some feel about being observed by colleagues, this can exacerbate the problem, hence the less dramatic invitation to take the 'chair'.*

Learning Purpose

The purpose will vary across the age-range from post-school nursing and medical students to experienced practitioners practising appraisal, performance interviewing or introducing new techniques – end-of-life care, for example

The primary purpose may be clinical or interpersonal but with an SP, communication skills will usually dominate.

For the purposes of this book I have adopted the definition of 'clinical skills' formulated by the Yorkshire and the Humber NHS in their *Clinical Skills and Simulation Strategy* of August 2010: 'Any action performed by staff involved in direct care of patients which impacts on clinical outcomes in a measurable way and includes:

- Cognitive or thinking skills such as clinical reasoning and decision making – *involves talk with patients*

- Non-technical skills such as team working and communication – *involves talk with colleagues and patients*

- Technical skills such as clinical examination and invasive procedures – *involves talk with patients.*

According to this definition all learning purposes will be concerned with some aspects of clinical skills, whether directly or, indirectly, as with appraisal interviewing.

- All SPs should be aware of the learning purpose and the training or professional level of the learners.

- Feedback should be attuned to learning level and purpose.

- It is worth remembering that the learning purpose may be concerned with collecting research data, piloting best ways to use SPs, or team training incorporating interpersonal concerns.

- The learning purpose can be made secure with an appropriate choice of a supporting 'framework' or visual display, to provide insights and reminders while interacting with the SP.

- While the content of a session may be clear – let's say it's about negotiating a treatment plan with the patient – it is equally important to plan how this will be achieved. The maxim: *awareness, understanding, and application* provides sound cover for any learning plan involving an SP. As can be seen in the charts below (taken from Bloom's *Taxonomy of Educational Objectives*). Though the maxim is simple to apply, it has profound underpinning.

Cognitive Domain Categories

• Knowledge	Awareness
• Comprehension	Understanding
• **Application**	Application
• Analysis	
• Synthesis	
• Evaluation	

Example of sub-skills

COMPREHENSION

- Understanding   information
- Grasping meaning
- Translating knowledge to new context
- Interpreting facts, comparing and contrasting
- Grouping facts – ordering
- Predicting consequences

Opportune Learning

This descriptor 'opportune learning' is not in common use. It reflects those occasions when something crops up that is not a predictable element of the learning purpose. In day to day life it is often referred to as 'going off at a tangent'. But an experienced facilitator may recognise an issue of professional value. Let's take the case of an avuncular patient in consultation with a young doctor or nurse (who doesn't look old enough to practise). The SP is being insensitively dominant, and the facilitator recognises an example of 'parent–child' behaviour, i.e. an example of transactional analysis as described in *Games People Play* by Eric Berne. This might provide an opportune learning moment. Whether to digress will depend upon matters of time, group maturity, continuity of group learning and such like. But it can provide a timely insight, if handled appropriately!

- Common culturally misunderstood phrases exemplify necessary and easily dealt with opportune moments – the story of the nurse who took an elderly patient wanting to *'spend a penny'* to the hospital shop, for example, but things can get out of hand if the temptation to unearth similar anecdotes is followed.

- It is common for certain phrases, introduced as illustrations of good consultation practice, to be used *formulaically*. For example, checking understanding by using the phrase, 'What will you tell your husband/wife when you get home?' Using formulaic language can be seen as being patient insensitive or more seriously, being clinically formulaic.

- The words *complicated* and *complex* are rarely deconstructed – and they need to be. Complicated processes of thinking are linear and, to an extent, predictable, whereas complex thinking is unpredictable. Clinicians use both processes, particularly when the patient, in a patient-centred interaction takes the lead thereby introducing complexity. A well-informed clinician will recognise what is happening – it doesn't take long to explain!

- All SP focused learning has a clinical background but, brief comments apart, it is not normally used for imparting clinical information. The Organ Donation workshop described in Part Two, with its multiple learning processes, is an exception.

It's a curious fact that we seem able to 'draw down' real emotions even when the reason for them is fictitious, right up to crying real tears. On one occasion I was in a flood of tears, including a snotty nose, and thought that dealing with an older man would be a challenge for the young woman in front of me. It was no -problem, she worked in a hospice where the likes of me were an everyday occurrence. SP – MS

Feedback

Example of SP Feedback rules

- Check if feedback is required in or out of role or both

- Focus on observed behaviour, not the person

- Focus on what is seen and felt (immediacy)

- Focus on description rather than judgement (no value judgements)

- Focus on specific behaviours in the context they occur

The feedback rules apply to all concerned. It's the facilitators' job to see that they are observed. Openly shared constructive feedback is a potent learning force, though facilitators often have to constrain and correct value statements of the *'I thought it was good'* variety. While value statements may be reassuring, they have little learning value. There are usually a series of feedback occasions during a session as different people take the chair.

- The quality of feedback provides a measure of organisational feedback for the facilitator and to a lesser extent for the SP. Does the case and its presentation fit the learning purpose, for example?

- The session's final, summary feedback is an occasion for reflection: What have you learnt today? What will you do differently tomorrow?

Metacognition

Know What You're Doing

Metacognitive factors: Self-reflection, the practice of inspecting and evaluating one's own thoughts, feelings and behaviour; and insight, the ability to understand one's own thoughts and feelings and behaviour, are central to the regulation of behaviours.

Readiness for self-directed change in professional behaviours: factorial validation of the 'Self-reflection and Insight Scale', Roberts C and Stark P, Medical Education 2008

The purpose of *metacognition* (yes – I know it's a word from another world) is to recognise what's going on in any learning situation, in order to respond and adjust. Two ideas may help underline the importance of this kind of thinking.

The practice of medicine, of health care in general, can be considered a craft. Experienced craftsmen and women, sculptors, engineers, actors, rarely have to think what to do next; they *know*. A sculptor, faced with a chunk of stone, will have an idea what it will look like before picking up a tool – and that only comes from long experience. But, 'knowing' accumulates from unique, individualistic personal experience. Which in turn depends upon understanding generated by past experiences. So, ideas do have a part to play in day-to-day experience beyond the initial analytical stage, when they are first introduced and practised.

Unfortunately, no-one can tell you what to do in unpredictable circumstances. Group learning is endemically unpredictable. There may be a degree of comfort in appreciating that 'knowing what to do' is classified as *practical knowledge* which is a 'craft' type skill unique to SPs and those facilitators who work with them. To that extent expertise, though helped by ideas from theory, can only grow through experience.

Learning ideas that may help with planning and reflection in Group Learning Contexts

Please note:

- The four learning contexts in the diagram below should initially be regarded, for practical reasons, at the level of awareness, e.g. group work seating should be arranged so that everyone can see and participate equally – self-evidently experiential learning depends upon ensuring the experience is instructive if not challenging – reflection 'on' as distinct from 'in' action requires dedicated time.

- Deeper understanding of the educational issues involved is only required by those educators who specialise and have continuity of group responsibility.

- The four chosen learning contexts are not exclusive influences. Workplace and ethnic cultural factors may have influence on learning outcomes, as may some socio-psychological issues.

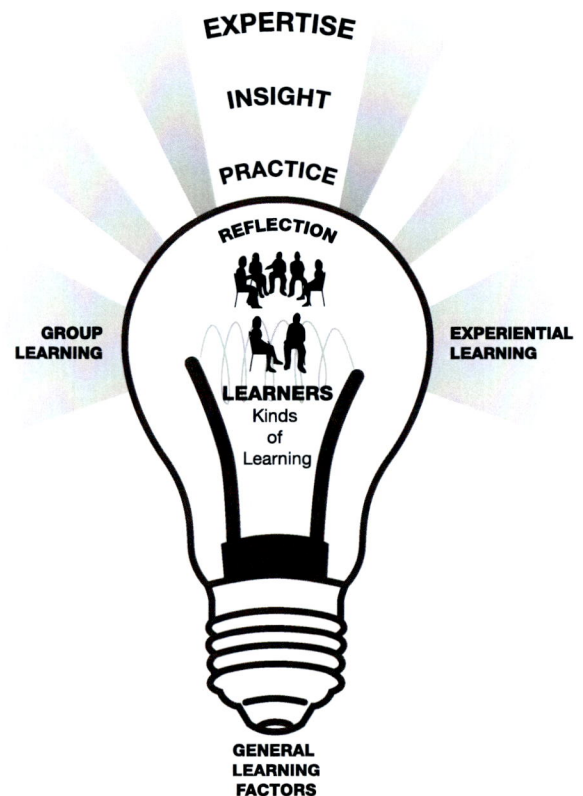

EXPERTISE

INSIGHT

PRACTICE

REFLECTION

GROUP LEARNING

EXPERIENTIAL LEARNING

LEARNERS
Kinds of Learning

GENERAL LEARNING FACTORS

General Learning Factors

> Readiness
> Gaining and Giving Attention
> Reinforcement
> Demonstration and Modelling
> Evaluating

Readiness

For us, readiness comes in two forms. The first concerns *mood;* is she or he in a suitable frame of mind to participate. The second concerns the possible gap between the group learning purpose and individual members' stage of learning. It's the difference between someone's unpreparedness having just come off a night on call and 'talking above someone's head', i.e. awareness of prior learning levels.

• Having no previous experience of acting out in the presence of peers makes some people very vulnerable. This form of readiness needs checking routinely.

• Floundering while in the chair can indicate lack of readiness. If and when this happens, ask for honesty: *Are you struggling?* Following on with a well-informed recap and opportunity to have another go can reap rewards for all concerned. It can preserve the self-esteem of the person in the chair as well as demonstrating an aspect of facilitator 'authority'. And, of course, discussing it with peers can solve the clinical problem at the heart of the flounder. It's always good to achieve more than one thing at a time!

Gaining and giving attention

Quality of attention is one of the most influential factors in active learning. Can you hear your school teacher saying, *QUIET* in a firm voice. Or, more plaintively, *listen please*. It's a universal problem! Active learning in a group depends to a high degree upon watching, noticing and listening. Non-verbal behaviour exchanges in a consultation can easily be missed if attention is not 100%.

• It helps to explore the learning purpose as you would a draft job description – the purpose needs to be internalised by the learners as a sounding board for immediate responses.

• The quote below from *Intelligent Kindness* by Ballat and Campling expresses a more profound use of attention:

'[There is] strong evidence, from research and patient experience that attentive kindness builds the sort of relationship between staff and patients within which reduction of suffering, increased trust, better communication, better understanding and diagnosis, and better cooperation make effective care more possible, and more likely'.

Reinforcement

Any therapeutic skill, if not consolidated by continual use, will wither, and if it involves important clinical application, it will require retraining. While there may be more latitude with interpersonal skills, they too can be treated too casually and wither. I've had personal experience of this as an SP in training undergraduate medical students in the use of summary. Later I spent numerous occasions as an SP in simulated surgeries. The surgery is organised for eight postgraduate doctors who consult with eight SPs in rotation at 10-minute intervals. It is (was) a high-stake assessment for certification to practise as a GP. Consulting with eight doctors in the same role, I became aware over time that summary was not often used. So I started counting. Thereafter, I never counted it being used by more than two doctors in each surgery. Curious, because summary achieves three things at once: it shows you're listening, gives you time to think and allows the patient both to check the correctness of your summary and provide an opportunity to review what they have said. Such a valuable skill needs constant reinforcement.

- The process of group learning with an SP is ideal for reinforcement. Observers can be asked to identify specific skills or behaviours which can then be reinforced during feedback. Experienced SPs can help reinforcement of interpersonal skills in their feedback: 'I did become aware of the long silence but it helped me to remember ...'

- While conforming to feedback rules, brief favourable comments by facilitators identifying details of good practice can sometimes be taken as praise, a powerful reinforcer.

- Eventually, reinforcement leads to that happy situation where you 'know' what to do without thinking – the province of the expert.

Demonstration and modelling

Used sparingly, if consultations are getting stuck, the facilitator can, on a 'let me have a go' basis, demonstrate a possible solution. Such an intervention can be timely. It can remove confusion, 'Oh I see now' (light-bulb moment), without undermining facilitator neutrality.

In my experience demonstration is rarely used, possibly because there is a conceptual conflict between leaving trainees to learn for themselves and associated facilitator reticence. Sometimes a demonstration can outclass lots of words.

Modelling is slightly different. A group member may model an aspect of good practice which needs to be highlighted as such and possibly reinforced during feedback. Modelling normally involves the unspoken imitation of sound practice picked up on a day-to-day basis. In a group learning context, model practice can be made explicit.

Modelling behaviour is most applicable to facilitation of group processes. Facilitators adopt a neutral role in order to encourage group members' viewpoints. They suppress their own opinions. They try to ensure everyone participates constructively. Behaving like this they model the fact that the learners' interest is paramount and by the same token that group members are largely responsible for their own learning.

- Facilitators need to signal if they feel it important to change their customary behaviour with a phrase such as, 'I wouldn't normally do this but …' This could be the case if they felt a demonstration would reveal good practice more effectively in the time available.

Evaluating

Identifying the learning accretion from any situation is essential. The quickest and cheapest way to achieve this is by simply observing what happens and making a subjective response. Other ways range from a filled in sheet at the end of a session to full scale academic research.

- The quality and range of feedback provides evidence of some learning outcomes. For example, do the responses reflect a superficial level of observation or evidence of deeper thought?

- It should be remembered that while we, as SPs, facilitators and participants, become deeply engaged in discrete aspects of professional practice, we rarely know whether it is translated into everyday behaviour. Interpersonal behaviour change is difficult to measure. Results at the humanistic end of the simulation spectrum are far less predictable than those at the high-tech, clinical skill end.

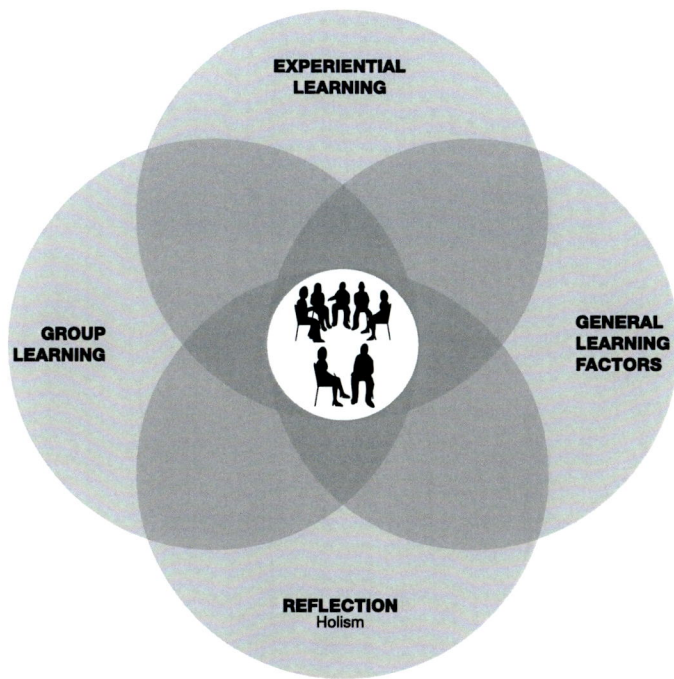

Experiential Learning

At the heart of all learning is the search for meaning in experience

Alan Rogers, *Teaching Adults*, 1996

Self-determination theory identifies three innate needs that allow us to have optimal function and growth throughout life: autonomy, competence, relatedness. Put another way, we want to be in tune with ourselves and be recognised as such by others; to be in control of our own lives in terms of our potential, drives and emotions; to be connected to others in a mutually caring manner. Self-determination theory also explores our intrinsic and extrinsic motivation to achieve. In crude terms: does it 'pay' us to learn, do we enjoy learning for its own sake, or do we manage to combine both?

The theory is very influential among health educators who assume practitioners will take responsibility for their own professional development. To that end, group work in the third year of Leicester Medical School is designed to foster independent group learning. The new Graduate Medical School in Derby has been built with team rooms furnished with computers

to embed self and small group independent learning. While the necessity for individual learning may be paramount, this potentially laissez-faire approach does pose problems for those without a strong commitment. For them, the ultimate forfeit is failure to gain a certificate to practise. It also tends to exclude even small inputs of didactic learning that may assist metacognition (there it is again). That said, the assumption that professional learners are autonomous, particularly at postgraduate level, provides a sound educational sub-text to experiential learning.

Historically, several powerful ideas have been subsumed into the phrase 'experiential learning'.

1. Interest in its power began as a reaction against the imposition of knowledge and the dominance of rote learning. *Prior experience* became thought of as the basis for most learning. Within that experience the role of affective as well as cognitive learning became recognised.

2. It was *found to be useful* for interpersonal encounters of various kinds, particularly for teasing out organisational problems, i.e. because it is dynamic and progresses from one experience to another. Academics have formulated experiential cycles that go, for example, from concrete experience to critical reflection, to thinking how to adapt, to trying out more proficient ways of working and then back again to concrete experience.

3. People react to experience in different ways, with distinct kinds of *learning styles*. Kolb (Experiential Learning, 1984) lists four. Which one, or combination of styles fits you?

Convergers tend to prefer abstract ideas and experimentation. They are good at problem solving, decision making and the practical application of ideas. Emotional expression and involvement with social and interpersonal issues is not their forte.

Divergers tend to be imaginative and able to regard life from many different points of view. They are good at conjuring up alternatives and responding to the feelings of others.

Assimilators are good at theorizing and making sense of disparate events and ideas. They tend to be inward looking, reflective, and they search for correct answers – their focus is on ideas rather than people.

Accommodators like to do things and get involved in new experiences. They will adapt on a trial and error basis to complex and unclear situations. Though they are said to be at ease with people they are sometimes seen as impatient and pushy.

> Honey & Mumford identify four styles with self-explanatory titles
>
> **Activist - Reflector - Theorist - Pragmatist**

When there is sufficient continuity of group membership and people are at ease with each other, facilitators will be able to recognise some of these characteristics.

- Experiential learning should be thought of as a process whereby ideas, attitudes, and skills derived from and continuously modified by experience are obtained. Whether that process leads to behaviour change is a step further on.

- Group learning with SPs is an active process which is not the case with all experiential learning. Beware, active learning as we practise it, is not the same as 'Active Learning' which is a discrete practice with its own methodology (see Reg Revens on Google).

- Experiential learning is an approach within which all concerned are obliged to find out how best to gain benefit – for themselves and others. In groups, it increases the potential to benefit by collaborative effort.

> *Simulation training sessions, which are structured with specific learning objectives in mind, offer the opportunity to go through the stages of the experiential cycle in a structured manner and often combine the active experiential components of the simulation exercise itself with a subsequent analysis of, and reflection on the experience, aiming to facilitate incorporation of changes in practice. Simulation offers the opportunity of practiced experience in a controlled fashion, which can be reflected on at leisure.*
>
> Ruth Fanning and David Gaba, *The Role of Debriefing in Simulation-Based Learning, Simulation in Healthcare,* Vol 2/2 2007

Learning in a Group

Working in groups requires three skills: an understanding of theory, knowledge of its application, and a trained experience in its use.

Josephine Klein, *Working with Groups*, 1961

Josephine Klein goes on to say that theory is only of use if it is *operational*, i.e. concerned with *how* theory is used. Happily for us, no theory underpins the group approach in the same way as experiential learning. If we assume that an experienced SP will know what is expected in the group setting, we can consider operational factors by questioning what is demanded of facilitators and group members in their efforts to get the best out of learning activity.

Selection of Member Tasks

- Contribute to a warm, accepting, non-threatening climate
- Approach learning as a cooperative activity
- Accept that the purpose of the group is professional learning
- Participate in a discursive manner
- Share the leadership of learning
- Accept distributed tasks and provide associated feedback
- Be prepared to try things out and make mistakes
- Be prepared to challenge colleagues to establish meaning

Derived from Learning Thru Discussion by WM Fawcett Hill, 1962

Selection of Sessional Facilitator Tasks

Preparation for and with group

- Check practicalities, e.g. room booked?
- Discuss case potential and process with SP
- Establish learning stage of group – prior learning?
- Introduce or revise group and SP procedural rules
- Agree learning focus

Managing the task

- Distribute tasks – interviewer's agenda, observer roles etc
- Ensure maximum engagement – rotate tasks
- Stop ^ Start – with in-depth discussion/feedback
- Relate final session feedback to learning focus

Reflection

- Leave time for silent personal reflection on 'what's learnt'

We need no long description to imagine how difficult it may be for a facilitator faced with a participant who doesn't participate:

How many reasons why? What solutions are there? What about group members watching how it's dealt with?

Conversely, how might a participant feel who has been unfairly criticized by a colleague in front of colleagues? The group is a person-to-person dominated arena requiring clarity of purpose, mutuality of engagement, which, if it is skilfully handled by all concerned, can result in worthwhile outcomes not available with other methodologies.

Responses (no help offered here) may involve high level thinking, feeling and behaving capabilities.

Skill is built up by doing it; by getting involved.

There is plenty of analytical advice regarding group function but very little advice as to how to implement the tasks listed above in what is known as the *group dynamic*. If you haven't already guessed, this is:

> *The combined configuration of mental, emotional and physical energy in the group at any one time and the way this configuration undergoes positive* and negative* change.*
>
> **positive = task orientated, process orientated, expressive, interactive, confronting, personal work orientated and charismatic.*
>
> **negative = alienated, culturally restricted, psychologically defensive.*
>
> John Heron, *The Complete Facilitators Handbook*, 1999

Holistic Learning

Key to holistic thinking is the attention it pays to experiential learning, to relationships and human values. The term is used across disciplines to represent a wider, more complete view of how things and people relate. An archaeologist looking at recovered pottery will want to know how it was made (skills), what sort of society it was made in (anthropology), maybe why it was made (practical, spiritual) and so on.

> *A holistic approach is about the ability to understand and respect the values, culture, family beliefs and structure, and understand the ways in which these will affect the experience and management of illness and health.*
>
> Competence No 6, The RCGP Curriculum: Introduction and User Guide, 2012

The quote above indicates that holistic learning relies deeply upon humane thinking as its purpose – and is regarded as a competence. Experiential group work with SPs aspires to be holistic in different ways:

Firstly, there need be no content boundaries to any discussion between group members, between facilitators and the patient matters identified, as long as they have some relevance to the learning focus. For example, a significant number of patients report with work related stress which may cover a multitude of background situations and possible causes – interest in and consideration of the workplace can be important for treatment considerations.

Secondly, we've touched upon the idea of the whole person while considering self-determined learners. While not necessarily dealing with this 'person' during group sessions it is important to regard and respond to group members in a holistic manner – people's life experiences and values may well emerge as issues in the discussion.

Thirdly, the Royal College of General Practitioners (RCGP) requires GPs to be *patient-centred* and *holistic* in their day-to-day work. This requirement embeds the importance of *triple diagnosis*, i.e. a diagnosis that includes a wide interpretation of physical, social and psychological factors. While medical students may take this as axiomatic, applying it in the real world can be problematic for a host of reasons – issues of clinical uncertainty, patients' reluctance to disclose intimate matters, to name but two.

At one level this entails obtaining a patient history that is complete, in that it takes into account the patient's *lifeworld*. To explore this, we created the case scenario of a middle aged woman who, having previously been diagnosed and treated for work-based stress, returned to the doctor two weeks later to say that she wanted to stop taking the medication – medication that is only effective if taken for four weeks and more. It transpired that the woman's mother strongly disapproved of pill taking – vital information that enabled the doctor to negotiate the next step on the basis of (holistic) information from the patient's *lifeworld*.

1. Eliciting a holistic history involves a high level of interpersonal skill. Sometimes this is matched by a clinical uncertainty that calls for honesty and negotiation with the patient.

2. For the SP, the above scenario calls for some subtle judgements. As a general point, how difficult do you make it for the doctor to find out about your dominant mother? More specifically, do you shut out a doctor with whom you have little affinity? Do you include little cues for the doctor who creates rapport? What will persuade you to take the medication?

3. There are a number of learning issues for the facilitator to follow up: ethical – does this woman need to face up to her mother and will you help her; clinical – regarding alternatives to medication or acceptance of no treatment; interpersonal – the person-to-

person relationship and skills required to get a complete holistic story.

4. The importance of a holistic approach should form an explicit sub-text in all such episodes.

Reflection

Reflection must be inextricably connected with experience if the experience is to have any value. Expertise regression is not unknown amongst those who refuse to challenge their own actions. Critical thinking implicitly underpins reflection. Our reflective purpose is to find ways in which experience can, over time, drive higher-order practice.

Selecting ideas from the 'reflective practice' literature helps us distinguish between thinking on the job and thinking afterwards; thinking *in* practice and thinking *on* practice. We've already floated the idea that practical knowledge cannot be codified (collected and organised into a system). But more positively, Argyris and Schön and others have introduced the idea of *theories in use* to describe how individual practitioners do unpack their actions *in* practice using their own micro-theories. These are sometimes called maxims, heuristics or rules of thumb. They accrue over time from experience. That's fine, but how do theories in use develop over time in such a way that expertise grows? Using the Dreyfus derived language from 'novice to expert', Bion and his colleagues asked similar questions. So what turns experience into learning and why do some benefit more than others? The answer is the reflective process, a complex activity 'in which both feelings and cognition are closely related and interactive'. Schön calls individuals who engage in this activity *reflective practitioners*.

Learning and the role of reflection in learning do not seem to be as tidy as the experiential learning cycle suggest.

Jennifer Moon, *Reflection in Learning & Professional Development*, 1999

Reflective practitioners 'reconstruct experience in a continuing and pervasive manner' in several different, often untidy ways. One such collective way is integral to SP resourced group work in the customary feedback procedure – what went well? – what could have been done differently? – what did the observers witness? – what alternatives might be tried? And so on. Individual reflection can be further grounded using the frameworks employed to promote experiential learning. The Leicester Assessment Package (LAP) or Calgary-Cambridge provide examples of validated frameworks against which to bounce ideas. Practitioners can invent their own reflection criteria. We devised a framework for GP registrars to practise achieving concordance with patients. Sounding boards can be simple or complex. The learning focus for the day can double as a ready-made sounding board.

> *The concept of reflection on an event or activity and subsequent analysis is the cornerstone of experiential learning experience. Facilitators guide this reflective process.*
>
> Ruth Fanning and David Gaba, The Role of Debriefing in Simulation-Based learning, Simulation in Healthcare, Vol 2/2 2007

Achieving Patient Concordance

A Framework for Action

ICEE + CRENA

- Include patient's ICEE
- C - Present treatment choices
- R - Explain risks
- E - Provide evidence re-choices
- N - Negotiate patient's preferred options
- A - Agree action plan

- Suitably chosen frameworks can be used for on-the-spot reflection.

- Reflection on action can be structured in if there is continuity of group membership and facilitation.

- Longer-term reflection requires setting aside a short time at the end of a session. Silent thinking about a single issue, or about what's happened more generally, can be very useful if thoughts are then shared across the group.

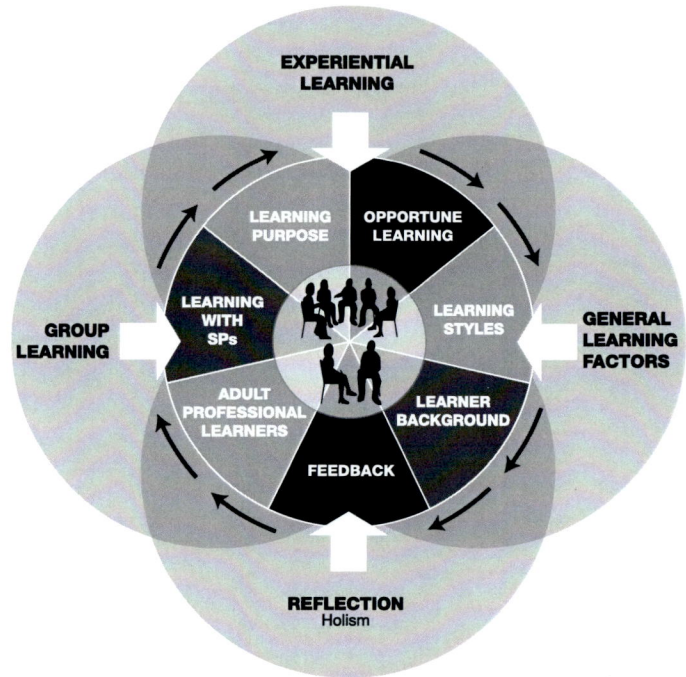

> *Medical simulation can help achieve important goals in medical education that have become increasingly difficult to address. Rooted in adult learning theory, simulation can effectively meet the needs for adults to be active learners, to learn in relevant contexts, and to individualise their own learning plans. By compelling reflection both during and after the exercise, simulation training fosters reflective practice.*
>
> Huang GC, Gordon JA, Schwartzstein RM, Millenium Conference 2005 on Medical Simulation: A Summary, Simulation in Healthcare, Vol 2

Chapter Five

Interpersonal Skills

'...there is growing evidence of a link between good interpersonal skills and health outcomes'

Greco M, Brownlea A, & McGovern J,
Impact of patient feedback on the interpersonal skills of general practice registrars: results of a longitudinal study, *Medical Education*, 2001; 35

It is helpful to consider interpersonal skills as three interdependent consulting elements.

Skills

The skills enable us to identify and discuss what needs to be done. They provide one level of feedback language for what happens.

Behaviours

Behaviour drives what happens. Behaviour can be analysed in terms of its composite skills and ways in which it may be modified by relationships.

Relationships

Interpersonal behaviour is endlessly variable and fascinating. The context concerns how it affects professional behaviour and the consequent health outcomes.

The Professional Context

- Interpersonal skills are integral to the application of clinical expertise

- Interpersonal skills provide the content for most action learning with SPs

- Clinical content is woven into SP case-based interaction

- Interpersonal skills in healthcare can only be acquired through practice

- Learning from practice requires the three elements of interpersonal skills language for reflection

Interpersonal Skills

Contexts

Interpersonal skills are used **socially** in all healthcare situations

Interpersonal skills are used **professionally** by doctors, nurses and health workers on a one-to-one basis with patients at home, in hospital and at their most extended, in GP surgeries

Inter-professional talk in surgical team work – given the need for attention to hand-eye skills, monitors and multi-person coordination in exacting circumstances – is integrated and referred to separately as **Human Factors**

Interpersonal skills are used in various ways according to clinical circumstance. Duty of care and respect is subsumed whatever the manner of use.

Dilemma

The acquisition of interpersonal skills in medicine poses problems for medical educators. As will be seen below, there is a long list of skills and a complicated connection with the way they are played out as behaviours with patients. This raises the curricular question of how best to introduce and practise them. The problem is compounded by the inevitably parallel task of imparting clinical knowledge and skill. In student and registrar minds the clinical imperative frequently crowds out the interpersonal. Different approaches to the problem are illustrated in the Part Two descriptions of SP use at Leicester Medical School and the University of Nottingham Graduate Entry School. A novel approach was piloted at the University of Saskatchewan, College of Medicine, where students were first introduced to patient-centred communication using a Lego model of the patient's story in a role-play, i.e. without clinical content. [1]

[1] Read more in Using a Lego-Based Communications Simulation to Introduce Medical Students to Patient -Centred Interviewing, Rutledge Harding S and D'Eon F, Teaching and Learning in Medicine 13(2) 130-135, 2001

The Language of Interpersonal Skills

Identifiable single skills most used in healthcare

Questioning

Closed questions	*Reply determined questions*
Open questions	*Open response invited*
Echo question	*Response repeated as a question*
Probing questions	*A search for deeper or extended meaning*
Proposal questions	*Closed-cum-open questions requiring discusson*

Listening

Hearing	*Registering what is said (distinct from just listening)*
Acknowledging	*Reply confirming what's heard*
Use of silence	*Indicates listening or waiting to encourage additional disclosure – a way of switching control*

Responding

Answering	*Giving a verbal or non-verbal reply*
Affirming	*Indicating importance and/or agreement with a response*
Listening noises	*Ums – errs – sucking teeth etc. – (**N**on-**S**pecific **P**rofessional **N**oise)*
Parking	*Item of patient agenda to be dealt with later*

Informing

Informing	*Providing new knowledge*
Explaining	*Adding meaning to new or existing knowledge*
Chunking	*Sequencing and limiting the amount of information given (using lay language)*
Checking	*Establishing information or explanation is understood*

Summarising

Summary	*Shortened review of what's been discussed*

Signalling

Signalling	*Sharing of doctor/nurse intentions with patient (transitional statements in USA)*

Empathising

Empathising	*Affective or cognitive understanding of what's in the patient's mind*

Non-verbal

Non-verbal	*Covers bodily movement, facial expression and tone of voice*

N.B. This is only a list of the most commonly used professional skills

---

Eye Contact

The eyes are usually considered to be the principal means by which man gathers information. However important their function as 'information gatherers', we should not overlook their usefulness in conveying information. For example, a look can punish, encourage, or establish dominance. The size of the pupils can indicate interest or distaste.

Edward T Hall, *The Hidden Dimension*, Anchor Books, 1969

Non-Verbal Communication e.g. Hand Talk
The hand waves, salutes, applauds, greets, insults, indicates helplessness or surrender or despair, threatens, interrogates, informs. These are its telecommunications.

Raymond Tallis, *The Hand*, 2003

Interpersonal Behaviours

Interpersonal behaviours are composed of more than one interpersonal skill.

It is ever variable behaviours that play a vital role in professional practice.

Health professionals need to learn these skills, SPs need to recognise them.

A Patient Story

Interpersonal skills and behaviours cannot be used in the abstract: they need purpose. In everyday practice this involves real patient problems. The patient in this story has a problem but to illustrate the use of skills and behaviours, we also need a doctor agenda. Dr Garland has been on a consultation refresher course recently. She has come back wanting to try out three patient-centred prompts: 'starting anywhere' (being led by the patient); 'going there' (including the patient's background); and 'concordance' (negotiating a mutual agreement).

Consultation Expertise Model Framework (CEM)

STARTING ANYWHERE – GOING THERE - CONCORDANCE

On this occasion Dr Garland is accompanied by a Year 2 medical student called Ahmed, who, with permission might take part in the consultation. Ahmed has been introduced to clinical method, particularly the history taking part of it, together with SQITARS – the acronym for a checklist (framework) to help with questions about pain.

Clinical Methods Framework

HISTORY TAKING – EXAMINATION – DIAGNOSIS – MANAGEMENT

SQITARS Framework

Site – Quality – Intensity – Time - Arrows – Relief - Symptoms

Les Stretton is 61 years old. Two years ago he went to the surgery with neck pain and restricted movement. He was given a cervical collar and a prescription for Cocodamol. A month ago he returned with pain in his left hip. He was given an X-ray appointment, a 'fit' note that stated when he will be fit to work and told to continue with the Coodamol. He returns at the end of the month for the X-ray results. As an infrequent attender he sees a different doctor who only knows that he is a painter by occupation. By chance, the doctor has a Year 2 medical student with her.

. . . .

Dr Mr Stretton, isn't it? Please sit down. We haven't met but I gather you've been off work with hip pain. First of all, how do you like to be addressed? I'm Dr Garland and this is Ahmed, a medical student. Do I call you Mr Stretton, or Les? Which do you prefer? [professional *greeting* which will depend on tone of voice and facial expression for effect]

Les People at work call me Les.

Dr So, it's OK to call you Les [*n-v* sees Les nod]. Do you mind if Ahmed asks you a few questions to give him some practice? [n-v Les nods – Dr types, *patient not very expressive?* on record as a reminder]

Ahmed How long have you had this hip pain? [*closed Q*]

Les I'd had it a week or so before I came last time.

Ahmed Why do you think it happened? [*open Q*]

Les   I'm a painter and I spend a lot of time going up and down ladders and moving them from one place to another – it's easy to twist things. Maybe it's a sign of age – I'm not as nimble as I used to be.

Ahmed   *[nods – ums and har's – uses silence]* I need to ask you some medical questions about the pain to help Dr Garland – OK? *[signals intent - sees Les nod]* First of all, where exactly is the pain? *[closed Q - Les puts hand on left hip and prods]*. How would you describe the pain? *[open Q – Les looks puzzled]* Let me help – is it a sharp pain or dull, for example? *[suggestive closed Qs]*

Les   It's mostly when I move. It's not so bad when I'm sitting around at home.

Ahmed   How intense is the pain on a scale of 1 – 10? *[closed Q]*

Les   Depends. When I'm at work it can be 7 - 8, at home it's much less.

Ahmed   Does it go anywhere else? *[closed Q – negative nod]* When the pain is bad does it affect you in other ways?

Les   When I'm at work, it worries me. When I go up the ladder I wonder if I might not be able to get down. That's just one thing.

Dr   Thank you Ahmed, I'll carry on. Les, you said, 'That's just one thing'. What did you mean? *[mirror Q and picking up cue]*.

Les   Well it's not easy, is it? *[clue – no interruption]* There's all sorts of things *[pause]* What happens if I can't work again? I can't sit at home all day'. And *[… long pause..]*

Dr   And …. *[pause…echo Q]*.

Les   Well, the wife thinks I'm skiving – staying off work deliberately.

Dr   Why does she think that? *[open Q – eliciting patient's story]*

Les   I've no idea – she's a funny woman. Unless it's our Raymond.

Dr   Tell me about Raymond *[probing Q – 'going there']*

Les   Well, he's a bit funny, you know, a bit slow. Mind you, he's alright! She's looked after him – takes him to the Training Centre. I think she worries what is going to happen to him. But she doesn't talk to me much. She lives in a world of her own.

Dr   *[Nods– ummm]*. I can see it's really not easy for you *[empathy - pause]* Have I got this right? At 61 you are beginning to feel vulnerable at work, particularly with your painful hip, and life at home has become more tense than usual because you've been off work sitting around
[summary – empathic understanding - maintaining rapport]

SKILLED BEHAVIOURS

Greeting

•

Establishing

Rapport

•

Eliciting Patient

Story

•

Recognising

Cues and Clues

•

Maintaining

Rapport

•

'Going There'

•

Reassuring

•

Informing

•

Checking

Understanding

•

Negotiation

•

Concluding

Les   Yes. What will happen to our Raymond if I can't lift him? He thinks it a joke sitting on the toilet until I lift him off – always has. They might take him away. She's never needed a dog or a cat the way she's looked after him. And it's my responsibility to look after the both of them, isn't it?

Dr   Right, let's look at this one thing at a time [prioritising]. First, I don't think you need to be alarmist about Raymond. Nobody is going to take him away if he's been cared for the way you say [reassurance]. Now let's look at the X-ray – that's what you came for, isn't it? It does show wear and tear of your left hip. Now, given your age, this is not likely to change, but I think you can live with it if we give you some stronger painkillers and you're careful at work. What control do you have over the way the job's done? [informing – reassuring – open/probing Q]

Les   I'm the foreman but the real problem is the speed we're expected to complete jobs and to hit targets – I have to get the youngsters to read the paperwork sometimes.

Dr   It sounds like your job is just like mine [sharing - smile] Am I right in assuming you are worried about losing your job and money? [Les nods]. Medically, I can't turn back the clock about your hip but, given that you are careful with ladders and so on and use others to do some of the lifting and moving, you should have a few years yet. We can help with some pain killers. You might think it's not my business but I suggest you discuss your worries with your wife. What you think about that? [checking]

Les   My neck did get better over time, so maybe my hip won't get any worse. The painkillers haven't worked before – why now?

Dr   I get the sense that you're not a talkative chap. To what extent do you talk things over with your wife? [probing Q]

Les   Not much, she keeps things to herself.

Dr   Can I suggest you try to talk about the worries you've told me about and see what she says [proposal Q – negotiation]

Les   I'll give it a go.

Dr   Do we agree then – keep going – look after yourself at work – talk to your wife ? AND – come back in a month to tell me how things are going. Here's the prescription. [concluding]

Les   Thanks.

Reading between the lines it should be possible to see how a partial medical history was taken with the help of SQITARS to obtain a better understanding of the hip pain. In terms of CEM, the consultation did not 'start anywhere' until Dr Garland picked up the cue 'and', which took the consultation into the patient's lifeworld, thus 'going there' on a voluntary basis. There were elements of informing and negotiating at the end which verged into a concordant conclusion. Regarding concordance, do we know whether he will take the painkillers? He'd stopped taking the previously prescribed Cocodamol!

In a description like this we can't appreciate the effect of the doctor's eye contact, tone of voice or body language, which may well help turn any discrete interpersonal skill into effective clinical expertise.

Interpersonal Relationships

What health professionals say to patients, relatives and colleagues depends on the clinical purpose of the contact. How it is said depends upon the interpersonal skills and behaviours employed. How it is received, will depend upon unspoken 'vibes'. I'm not sure if that's the best word to describe an interpersonal feeling in an often fleeting professional relationship, but it will have to suffice. The vibes can significantly affect the way people react, irrespective of what is said. For example, some people are sensitive to being treated in an overly paternalistic manner. Similarly, new SPs are instructed to remove any prejudices they may have – for example, towards pregnant school girls, grossly overweight patients, foreign doctors, travellers, posh people.

More positively, impressions help us adjust our communication levels. In the example above, Dr Garland felt at one stage that Les was not very 'expressive'. We don't know whether this affected the way she related to him thereafter. We do know that smiles can have a powerful influence in rapport building but need using judiciously at funerals!

There is much insightful material in the published literature. The ego states, parent, adult, child and their variations introduced by Eric Berne (*Games People Play*) are part of consulting language: 'We must have an adult-adult conversation about this'. Patronising behaviour by a health professional might evidence a parent-child relationship. Whereas, 'Tell me what to do doctor', may be a patient adopting the 'child' state, or alternatively, evidence of a poor relationship, 'You're the doctor, you tell me what to do', if spoken assertively.

Interpersonal relationships are endlessly intriguing and may provide insights into professional situations. More practically, there are recurring circumstances when relationships affect the manner in which things are done. This is particularly the case with:

- Telephone consultations – when they go beyond the triage level and engage in the equivalent of a face to face consultation, there is a major problem. It is estimated that over 50% of the relationship is received non-verbally. The absence of this on the telephone necessitates behaviours that can be identified and taught.

- Inter-cultural consultations (working with interpreters is a speciality) depend upon knowledge of customary cultural demands. As this is usually partial, it is basic good practice to ask patients to make such sensitivities explicit.

- Breaking bad news – this 'moment in time' responsibility calls for a distinction between the way news is communicated about, for example, a chronic disease like epilepsy and a life threatening condition.

- End of life discussions – whether they are held in the community, the hospital or hospice – have become a specialist field with specific therapeutics, ethical, religious, and legal issues to be considered when conversing with potentially terminal patients.

Interpersonal skills and behaviours provide the strata upon which the clinical landscape is built.

English is the second language for many of the doctors we work with. This can lead to some curious relationship moments. Under a psychiatric role entitled, 'Morbid Jealousy' I present as an angry butcher who's seen his wife having lunch with another man. I use local dialect to some extent and tell the doctor how I've been hitting my wife, giving her a 'good pasting'; to which the response was, 'What's a good pasting?' On another occasion as the same angry butcher I was consulting with a doctor whose habit while thinking was to say, 'Oh yes – mm-yes – oh yes. I interrupted his thinking to explain how I'd been slapping my wife around to teach her a lesson. Then I said, 'You'd do that wouldn't you?' 'Oh yes – yes – mm-yes', was the reply.
SP – RF

The angry butcher anecdote illustrates how quickly SPs need to respond to maintain positive learning relationships. Second language learners present an additional dimension. Not knowing what a 'pasting' is can quickly be followed by, 'I hit er'. But the second occasion involves listening, an interpersonal skill issue, which may merit a time-out call by the facilitator.

Remember
Caring is catching

Frameworks

I have taken the liberty of referring to a range of helpful consultation procedures, checklists, models, structures, even acronyms, just part of the verbal jungle, as frameworks. Not to be confused with clinical procedures of course. Frameworks provide a learning resource, structure and memory support for the application of clinical knowledge and skill.

Rule of thumb – a rough and practical (individual) approach, based on experience

Checklist – list of items to be checked or referred to for comparison, identification or verification

Framework – a structured plan or basis of a learning approach

Interpersonal skills and behaviours are therefore, inextricably wedded to whatever framework(s) the health professional chooses. Often it is only a word or phrase that percolates through to the SP. For the record, what follows is therefore more akin to name dropping. It is in historical order to illustrate how current discourse contains an amalgamation of key words.

From way back
Clinical method adapted through the years with stage one, **history taking**, continuing to play a major training role using SPs and acting as the default mode when doctors pause mid-

consultation to ask themselves ,'Have I missed something?' i.e. not taken a complete history.

1957
Michael Balint, *The Doctor, his Patient & the Illness,* distinguishes between **illness** as suffered by the patient and **disease** as perceived by the doctor.

1984
Pendleton et al, *The Consultation: An Approach to Learning and Teaching*, is best known for **Pendleton's rules** which specify a now customary feedback procedure.

1986
The concept of patient-centred clinical method conceived by a group of Canadian doctors best known for **ICE(E** added later) – **I**deas, **C**oncerns, **E**ffects and **E**xpectations.

1987
Roger Neighbour's *The Inner Consultation*, 'en route' consultation checkpoints introduced the vocabulary of Connecting – Summarizing and the perhaps more frequently referred to, **Safety Netting** and **Housekeeping** (housekeeping concerns doctor wellbeing, particularly after psychologically disturbing cases).

1994
Leicester Assessment Package (LAP) provides a detailed means to analyse what is happening in a consultation. Condensed versions are used as a training framework.

1994
Greenhalgh and Hurwitz introduced the powerful notion of the patient **'narrative'** into the cannon of patient-centred consulting. Obtaining and sharing the patient's 'story' can require subtle interpersonal skills and behaviours.

1998
Skills for Communicating with Patients by Silverman, Kurtz and Draper together with the companion volume *Teaching and Learning*

Communication Skills in Medicine have been widely adopted as the basis for teaching programmes. SPs are likely to come across the acronym **ALOBA** (**A**genda-**L**ed **O**utcome **B**ased **A**nalysis). It is useful for SPs to be aware of the learning agenda of the person in the chair, in order to provide pertinent feedback that directly or indirectly assists consideration of the consultant's agenda.

2009

The Consultation Expertise Model in *Advanced Consulting in Family Medicine* contains the means to 'fingerprint' a consultation in eight domains. Designed for use by practitioners, the headings – *starting anywhere; going there; concordance* – can be used in practice as triggers for later reflection and accretion of consulting expertise.

It is important to note that all the above, and many other texts, have contributed to a unique understanding of good practice in community medicine. SPs and their facilitators play a small part in ensuring that this continues.

Insights

Most of what is written about 'communication skills' is concerned with advice and research about achieving safe clinical practice and skill assessment, i.e. the facilitator part of our mutual group learning activity. Our role as SPs is to represent patient cases that will prompt learning so we can give feedback based on what happens. To do this we need to be capable of recognising the skills

With time and experience all the skills and behaviours mentioned acquire extended meanings, often of a personalised kind.

Patient Disclosure Difficulties

- A belief that nothing can be done
- Reluctance to burden the doctor
- Not wishing to seem weak or pathetic
- Worry that fears will be confirmed
- Concern about relevance, e.g work

Example

Eliciting a behaviour that may require the creative use of several skills, can be hindered by the fact that an SP case may involve one or more of the disclosure difficulties listed in the above box. A challenge of this kind will provide the learner with an extended understanding of eliciting skills. Obtaining a complete history from a patient in denial is not easy. SPs need to recognise the extended challenge.

Example

Listening can have a variety of components. Do we, for instance, consider *hearing* to be a sub-skill of listening? Hearing can be broken down further – attending, understanding, remembering – and it carries the responsibility of appropriate silences, support, empathy and paraphrasing. There is also mindless listening which some interpret as hearing. Confusing! But, consider the SP statement, 'I was trying to listen but all I heard was your disinterest in what I want to say'. As an SP you didn't 'hear' that verbally, it came to you non-verbally. Even more confusing, but fun! An advanced example of extended meaning can be found in Simon Cocksedge's book, *Listening As Work in Primary Care,* Radcliffe, 2005.

Example

Paula Stillman, one of the first doctors to use SPs (standardised patients in the USA) talks about *signalling* as *transitional statements*. That is, statements by the doctor or nurse that share clinical intentions with the patient, e.g. 'I'll give you a prescription but <u>I need to know</u> whether you will actually take the pills'. Transitional statements are also implicitly more patient-centred because they *share* the doctor's agenda with the patient. Stick to the term *signalling* and you will be better understood this side of the Atlantic.

Beware one-dimensional practice of skills and behaviours

> *'it is dangerous to cultivate the notion of disembodied skills that exist independently of context and purpose.'*
>
> Michael Eraut, Developing Professional Knowledge and Competence, Falmer Press, 1994 p94

Interpersonal skills can be learnt mechanistically. Indeed, it is important to learn the full range of skills and the distinction between skills and behaviours, from the outset. But they must not be communicated like that. Formulaic use is insulting and a good way to fail professional exams. Checking patient understanding is good practice. That said, the phrase, 'What will you tell your husband/wife when you get home?' becomes a formulaic give-away if everybody simply repeats those exact words – as has happened.

Recognising patient-centred consulting

 A health worker who is also a parent can relate to a patient's concern with an ill child, for example. A doctor or nurse with psychology training may create a therapeutic relationship. Both are implicitly patient-centred. But these examples will only occur randomly. The issue of patient-centred v doctor-centred consulting needs to be recognised by SPs and facilitators. Putting aside those occasions when the medical agenda is paramount, a patient-centred approach goes way beyond questions of courtesy and respect to matters of 'holism' and safety.

Once SPs are aware of the distinction, it is not difficult to recognise the difference through our feelings – in everything the doctor has done or said, is she or he interested in me or only in solving my expressed medical problem? Patient-centred doctors will be communicating with patient feelings in a variety of ways: interest through eye contact, relating symptoms to lifestyle, open questions, signalling, silent listening, the list can go on. Crucially, does the doctor enter my 'lifeworld'? This is not just a patient feelings issue. The Royal Society of General Practitioners requires all GPs to be patient-centred for sound medical reasons.

If a consultation becomes *conversational*, it will usually be patient-centred. A conversational style makes disclosure easy and natural and, by definition, an adult-adult interaction. Multiple symptoms, anxiety or depression or family related problems, for instance, all require full clinical and lifeworld disclosure. A conversational style often denotes a skilled clinician, usually the result of long experience but, occasionally to be seen among trainees!

Recommended reading

Should the day come when simulation becomes a focus of study for SPs, Chapter 5 in *The Patient-Doctor Consultation in Primary Care: Theory and Practice,* by Jill Thistlethwaite and Penny Morris, RCGP, 2006 is a rewarding read –there are lots of extended meanings. And by the way, Penny Morris was one of the first in the UK to use actors to represent the 'patient voice' for training.

Afterthought

In the past there has been a lack of clarity about the relationship between clinical competence and interpersonal and communication skills. In my earlier experience there was still a tendency to regard their acquisition separately – often to be assumed of lesser importance given the volume of clinical skill and knowledge required. This dichotomy was addressed by a study published in 1999.

'On the one hand, it might seem that these two dimensions of clinical performance are independent, given that one is more cognitive, or knowledge based, and the other is more affective and interpersonal. On the other hand, the two dimensions also appear interdependent, in that interpersonal and communication skills would seem to be necessary for the operation of clinical competence and clinical competence would seem to be necessary to impart the confidence needed for interacting and communicating with the patient'.

J A Colliver et al,
Relationship between Clinical Competence and Interpersonal and Communication Skills in Standardised-patient Assessment, *Academic Medicine,* Vol 74/3 , 1999

The results showed clinical competence and interpersonal skills to be related – *in the context of the clinical encounter.*

This explains why, when talking about facilitation and simulation in the health world it should always be understood that any apparent separate consideration of interpersonal skills for learning purposes is always grounded in a clinical/health context.

Chapter Six

Feedback

Where experience and understanding come together

> *'Feedback is a must for people who want to have honest relationships. It connects us and our behaviour to the world around us.'*
>
> Chapter 7, The Skilful Art of Giving Feedback, *The Essential Handbook for GP Training* edited by Ramesh Mehay

Feedback can be one of those moments when a 'light-bulb' indicates a crucial insight; a moment when facilitator and simulator skills achieve meaning. More fundamentally, given that our focus is limited to observations of what happens with an SP, feedback lives out the Kolb learning cycle of: experience – reflection – theorising – action; all four stages of the cycle can happen during an SP group session.

Range of expectation

At one end of the spectrum, a new SP might give feedback based on the feeling responses experienced <u>as themselves</u>. At the other end, an experienced SP simulating a patient with significant life history and several chronic conditions will give feedback <u>as that patient</u>.

Where previous theorising comes together

Successful feedback depends upon:

- Authenticity and appropriateness of the patient case, or doctor/relative scenario

- Clarity of, and bonding with, the learning purpose – i.e. it fits the stage of learning.

- Nature of group composition and continuity – participants know what to expect.

- Facilitators' group management – positive mood achieved, tasks allocated etc.

- SP and facilitator feedback skill – both are well practiced.

- Observer feedback based solely on what is seen and heard – i.e. no value judgements.

The list indicates some of the many influential facets in play during a professional learning situation. Fortunately, the act of observed consultation so focuses attention that all else slips into the background. The foreground with its immediacy of action thereupon opens up the opportunity for single-minded feedback – only, of course **if elements in the above list are in place!**

It is worth noting that the number of variables in any SP group session will ensure that learning outcomes are unpredictable and can therefore be thought of as **emergent** *outcomes.*

Debrief – cf. – Feedback

Dictionary wise, the two words can seem to, and may sometimes overlap. But, they are used differently in clinical education. Debrief occurs at the conclusion of a simulated clinical activity involving several people, e.g. a simulated surgical operation. Human factors, which includes communication issues, is the appropriate title for activities preceding the 'debrief', which often includes a video of the participants in action as previously watched by observers.

What is feedback?

Feedback can be defined as 'specific information about the comparison between a trainee's observed performance and a standard, given with the intent of improving the trainee's performance'.

Bokken et al, Feedback by simulated patients in undergraduate medical education: a systematic review of the literature. *Medical Education* 2009; 43; 202-210

That's a skeletal definition from which one can almost smell the intention to assess students' performance. Feedback in the medical school is largely concerned with clinical performance. Work with SPs in a group setting concerned with feelings and the human condition requires something warmer!

Feedback can be described as giving someone information about how their behaviour is observed, understood and experienced.

From a Maasrtricht Medical School information sheet issued in April 2013, giving guidelines, conditions and rules for effective feedback

Though it does not bristle with the joys of human interaction, the Maastricht definition does express the purpose of feedback in a group setting with SPs. Feedback given to experienced community nurses is viscerally different from that given to GP registrars, veterinary students or prospective GP appraisers, but they all involve perceptions of the professional context. While predicated on behaviour change, feedback also involves confidence building and sustaining motivation in situations with multiple standards.

Maybe it's more helpful to look at the users' point of view. We know that participants appreciate feedback that is problem-centred, meaningful to their professional situation and immediately applicable. Frustratingly, there are always other factors. For example, feedback may well have a delayed application, so we need to regard it from the facilitator and SP viewpoint. Facilitators may feel something needs saying in support of future good practice. Qualifying factors and definitions apart, active learning situations with simulated patients provide a unique and potentially powerful opportunity to receive feedback from three informed sources: colleagues, SPs and facilitators. Of these, SP feedback should be unique and different.

Practicalities

A Reminder

Basic Feedback Rules for SPs

- Check if feedback required in or out of role or both

- Focus on observed behaviour, not the person

- Focus on what is seen and felt (immediacy)

- Focus on description rather than judgement (no value judgements)

- Focus on specific behaviours in the context they occur

Giving constructive feedback is a complex skill that grows with experience. For this first attempt, limit yourself to uncomplicated statements of feeling and only then if they are supportive, e.g. very neutrally, I was able to say all I needed to, or more positively, it was easy talking with you. Beware of making value judgements outside the role of patient, e.g. I thought you took a good history of my case. As a patient you would know nothing about medical history taking! Stick to making observations on what happened

Feedback Rules introduced in Chapter 2 continue to apply

In or out of role?

Before a session, it is standard practice for SPs to check whether facilitators want feedback in or out of role or both. While it may be appropriate for SPs to provide out of role feedback in those situations for which they have been trained as SP 'teachers', and the learning purpose is a discrete part of the student curriculum, out of role feedback raises important issues.

- SPs train to 'become' a patient and talk with the 'patient voice'. So authenticity is threatened when they move in and out of role.

- With patients who are totally consumed with their own concerns or in some way limited in their ability to give meaningful feedback, there is a difficulty. This can be overcome if the SP comes half out of role and speaks on behalf of the patient; 'Mrs T felt you understood her problem and didn't rush her', for example.

- Simulator educators need specific training and suitable learning situations to come in and out of role and still retain patient authenticity.

- While responding in role, experienced SPs may well have an interior monologue going on, i.e. silently registering their own opinion. This may contradict what they are engaged to feel and report on. Out of role it becomes difficult to keep such opinions buttoned-up. I have found this particularly difficult when simulating a doctor in a performance or appraisal interview (thankfully not my doctor).

I have felt uneasy whenever I've have given feedback out-of-role. It can feel like giving advice. Few health workers like receiving advice from lay people!

Giving Feedback in Role

Giving feedback in role is one of the SP skills usually left to SPs' discretion. But, expressing feelings about a consultation in the patient voice demands imagination and verbal dexterity. It is left to individual discretion because it is difficult to provide suitable training. You are left knowing what you have to do with little beyond an example to help. For example, your scenario indicates you are a 68 year old man who drinks 8 pints a night, has reduced his smokes to 10 a day and attends surgery with a urinary problem. After taking a detailed history the doctor says, 'You must stop drinking as of now'. How do you respond? 'OK doc' – 'You must be joking' – 'What'll happen if I don't?' – 'My missus has been telling me to do that for years'. But the feedback in role might be, 'I know I must give up me drinking but I would have welcomed some help – I have tried'.

What helps of course is how you've previously personalised the case so you can quickly respond in role.

Group process

Value-added feedback is contingent on the following agreed processes between SP and facilitator having been established with the group:

- The learning level and experiential history of the group is explicit – e.g. have they worked with an SP previously?

- The manner in which the facilitator chooses to work will be understood *by all*.

- The learning purpose and process will be understood and agreed.

- The session agenda source will be known and agreed – e.g. the group may have chosen the agenda; the agenda may be curriculum based within which the ALOBA framework may dictate that a student choses the agenda; the agenda may revolve around a chosen patient case which may be psychologically or assessment based. Feedback will attend to the agenda source.

- The feedback process may have a content frame such as LAP or the Calgary-Cambridge five stage model and/or a process frame such as Pendleton or SET-GO.

S.E.T. – G.O.

- What I **S**aw

- What **E**lse I saw

- What I **T**hink

Facilitator then gets group to:

- Clarify **G**oal

- Produce **O**ffers of how to get there

- Within the chosen framework the necessity to allocate observation tasks to group members will be known, for example, half the group members may be asked to identify and record the interpersonal skills used, while the other half register examples of a strategy, such as ICEE. Interpersonal skills can be split into verbal and non-verbal as an alternative. Very different agendas will arise with experienced practitioners.

- There may be personal feedback mid-session as participants follow each other as consultor, in addition to end of session feedback. This will also depend on the length of time devoted to a declared framework as used for reference and analysis.

Group receptivity

In the early stages of group development, participants may be uncomfortable receiving feedback from colleagues and facilitators. However, more intransigent problems can impede progress. One USA medical school set up a research study to deal with specific receptivity problems. They involved faculty to simulate the behaviour of students who: 1 - are shy and unassertive, 2 - dispute feedback, 3 - appear disinterested. This resulted in clearly defined strategies.

Halina Brukner et al., Giving effective feedback to medical students: a workshop for faculty and house staff, *Medical Teacher*, Vol. 21, No 2, 1999

Similar sensitivities are not uncommon with experienced practitioners in denial about quality elements of their habitual practice.

Facilitators are responsible for engendering a suitable mood for feedback. This is difficult to achieve without continuity of group membership, though it is not unknown for a facilitator to end up with an anarchic group after several sessions. To maximise learning, groups need to become exploratory, to go beyond listening and reflecting on feedback to trying out new approaches. Key to this is the need to make mistakes; to try new techniques; to stumble and try again; to make colleagues laugh and yet learn.

Happily, there are facilitators who only have to sit down in a group and the mood is heightened. Beyond the use of frameworks, adept facilitators will, for example, enable groups to deal with uncertainty, understand the meaning of patients' lives and simultaneously grapple with multiple points of view.

The key to effective feedback is to offer both challenge and support but the rules are often used as reasons to be supportive without being challenging.

David Pendleton et al, *The Consultation: An Approach to Learning and Teaching*, Oxford, 1994

Feedback process

This will vary from one facilitator to another and may vary according to the agenda. In my experience Pendleton's rules, whereby feedback is first requested from the person who's consulting, is commonly used to start the process.

My preferred start is a period of silence to scan observational notes and reflect on what's been seen. Locally, for specific workshops, such as ICEE and concordance, we ask the SP and consultor to write down their private thoughts – not to be disclosed until an appropriate moment.

The sequence between the four feedback sources can be varied. For instance, a skilled facilitator may concentrate on probing for in-depth meaning and challenging the feedback of others, rather than making a personal contribution. When the person consulting and the SP have noted their private thoughts, it is often revealing to elicit group feedback first.

To make best use of a recorded consultation all observers should be given a viewing purpose to ensure they note down specific behaviour and interpersonal skills.

For mid-session feedback it is very beneficial for the person consulting or a group member to try out alternative approaches on a short-time basis. With one core case this process may occupy a significant amount of session time.

It is my custom to allow time at the end of the final feedback for each member of the group – it may also involve the SP and facilitator – to reflect on what they have learnt on a simple form, as below, and exchange their reflections with the whole group. Colleague feedback can be very thought provolking!

**Interpersonal Skills Session
Leicester VTS 18/09/12**

Learning Capture Sheet

Reminder - Professional learning concerns an AWARENESS of the range of factors involved in a topic, sensitivity to personal levels of UNDERSTANDING and the ability and commitment to APPLY that learning in practice.

Individual Learning Points - Please write down what you have learnt 'personally' during the session, things that apply to YOU and nobody else, i.e. unpredictable, unintended learning.

Action Learning Points – Aspects of the session content which you will remember and absorb into your future consulting.

It is customary for checklist feedback to be given by SPs who consult with students alone, i.e. to previously known criteria – with recorded evidence as an impartial record. This is a specific practice which may involve the SPs leaving the room to reflect before going back to deliver the feedback, in or out-of-role. As far as I know, we have no experience of this practice in the East Midlands.

Feedback outcomes

The purpose of SP group work is learning as expressed in future professional behaviour. It is simulated experience and the episodic feedback on what happens – from three different sources – that is assumed to drive this learning. Outcome criteria derive from the quality of daily professional practice together with the aspirations embedded in the literature and training assessment processes. Tantalisingly, such logical outcomes are rarely apparent. For me the outcomes are sufficient if a session devoted to worthwhile aspects of practice is acted out positively, reflecting a feeling that health workers value engagement in activity related to their daily lives. Desired outcomes reside in future practice quality and high levels of assessment results, i.e. very fuzzy, difficult to measure outcomes.

If honestly given, the learning points from any one session will be as varied as the prior experience of the participants, perhaps with a few common points that come up in feedback reviews, such as, 'I should use summarising more'. The best outcome indicator, I suggest, is the quality of the feedback interchange. If that includes insights and perceptive observation, that's good!

End of session evaluations, in my experience, do tend to indicate approval ratings at the top end of the Likert scale.

There is little research evidence to show that SP group based learning leads to behaviour change, partly because of the difficulty of following through and identifying change, but largely because there is little sustained experience with SPs, apart from in medical schools. However, and it is a big however, there is a belief that it does cause behaviour change and there is partial evidence derived from real patient feedback that it can.

Findings showed that systematic patient feedback at regular intervals throughout GP training resulted in sustained levels of interpersonal skills.

… there is growing evidence of a link between good interpersonal skills and health outcomes.

Greco, Brownlea & McGovern, Impact of patient feedback on the interpersonal skills of general practice registrars: results of a longitudinal study, *Medical Education* 2001; 35: 748-756

Feedback outcomes might be more meaningful if participants followed this dictum:

'… however disorienting, difficult, or humbling our mistakes might be, it is ultimately wrongness, not rightness, that can teach us who we are'.

Kathryn Schulz,
Being Wrong: Adventures in the Margin of Error, 2010

Afterthought 1

CARE

Consultation and Relational Empathy

How was the doctor at:

1. Making you feel at ease
2. Letting you tell your story
3. Really listening
4. Being interested in you as a whole person
5. Fully understanding your concerns
6. Showing care and compassion
7. Being positive
8. Explaining things clearly
9. Helping you to take control
10. Making a plan of action with you

A specific outcome measure!

The CARE measure above provides a good general list of doctor attributes for SP feedback, as a back-up to any specific agenda focus arranged with the facilitator.

Taken from; Mercer et al, The consultation and relational empathy (CARE) measure: development and preliminary validation and reliability of an empathy-based consultation process measure. *Family Practice* Vol 21; No 6.

Afterthought 2

Feedback – example of an SP reminder list

- Find out the status of the group – undergrads – F1/2s – ST 1/2/3 – practitioner

- Establish with facilitator whether to give feedback in or out of role

- If asked, give feedback on certain aspects, i.e. 'use of open questions', stick to that

- Try to memorise statements/questions/NSPN by consultor to use as evidence

- Never make value judgements or give opinions, i.e. never, 'That was good'

- If giving feedback in role – stay as patient, i.e. 'I liked it when you asked about my daughter because …'

- Always remark on things observed

- Negative feedback can be prefaced by patient statements such as, 'I would have been happier if you weren't chewing gum'

- Use interpersonal skills language if giving feedback out of role

SP - EBW

Afterthought 3

Persistent Feedback Problems

One of the most important rules is to feedback using evidence of what has been seen and heard. Facilitators customarily ask observers to record what they see and hear, i.e. with specific detail, e.g. when you said, 'Can you explain that a bit more', the patient paused and shook his head (a significant moment?). Despite such instructions too many group members continue to use value judgements, which prompt little or no learning. It is worth repeating that working with SPs provides a clinically safe opportunity to try out alternative approaches; to test out different personal ways of doing things in a context of professional guidance.

Afterthought 4

Light-Bulb Moments in historical texts - an example

Time In – Time Out

Excerpted: page 43, from:

Howard Barrows, *Simulated (Standardised) Patients and other Human Simulations, A comprehensive guide to their training and use in teaching and evaluation.* Health Science Consortium, Chapel Hill, NC, 1987

An important technique in teaching with the SP is the 'time in – time out' technique. It is characteristically used in small-group learning but can be employed with larger groups of students. During the student-SP encounter, watched by the other students and the teacher, the teacher can call 'Time out' at any time and the SP is instructed to go into what can best be called suspended animation, acting as if he is no longer in the room. The teacher and the other students can probe the examining student's thoughts, ideas and strategies, find out what hypotheses are being entertained, how data from the patient is being received, and what the student plans to do next.

When the teacher, or a student in the group, says, 'Time out', the SP is instructed to no longer respond to any question, and should look away from the student to avoid any communication, even eye contact. The SP cannot laugh, show surprise, or express any evidence of awareness of the conversations or remarks made by the students or teacher. It is inevitable that students will look at the SP as they discuss their thoughts about the problem, symptoms, and signs presented by the SP. The SP cannot be seen out of role, looking like someone else, as this will destroy the impact of the simulation. This is why 'time in – time out' is best thought of as a state of suspended animation for the SP.

When someone in the group says, 'Time in, the SP must continue as if back in the room, from the point where 'Time out was said. However, the SP must not show any evidence of having heard any of the comments made during time out. He cannot be seen to anticipate any questions, instructions, or particular maneuvers or approaches that will be used by a student as the result of time out discussions.

 N.B. With practitioners, rather than students, time out may be used more flexibly, *because* **SPs can hear what is being discussed and therefore respond to test-out a learning suggestion.**

Developing Expertise _____

Finding new skills

Competence – the ability to do the job

Performance – the ability to do the job well

Expertise – a definition

Having a special skill, knowledge or judgment

Expert – a definition

Having *extensive* skill or knowledge in a particular field

Expertise levels

Levels used are those of the Dreyfus brothers

(Herbert & Stuart Dreyfus: The Power of Human Intuition and Expertise in the era of the computer, Free Press NY, 1986)

Novice – Advanced beginner – Competent – Proficient – Expert

[Novice and Advanced beginner levels are included in Basic Skills]

Expertise identification

Behaviours at each of three levels are illustrated by indicative statements, i.e. what can be seen and heard happening between SP and student, trainee or practitioner, from the point of view of the facilitator's or SP's skill

Expertise triangulation – expertise development to develop expertise!

Expertise development is the common factor in a three-sided interaction between the *learner* - (outcomes – professional behaviour development), the *facilitator* - (organization – -group management – feedback – learning) and the *SP* - (authenticity – responsiveness – feedback)

SP Expertise Development

Realistically and consistently presenting a role in the same way has been said to require both above-average intelligence and emotional maturity

Bowman et al, Improving the skills of established general practitioners: the long term benefits of group teaching, *Medical Education*, 26,1992

The attributes of simulated patient presentations can be regarded according to the following four domains

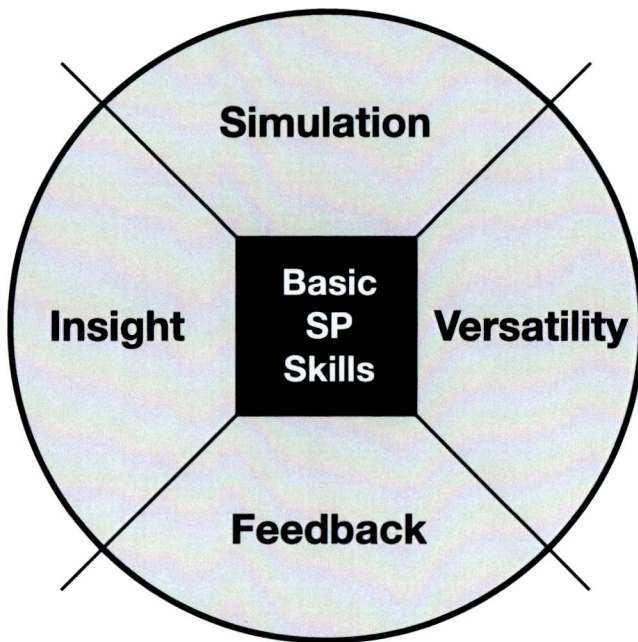

Within each domain three levels of expertise can be established

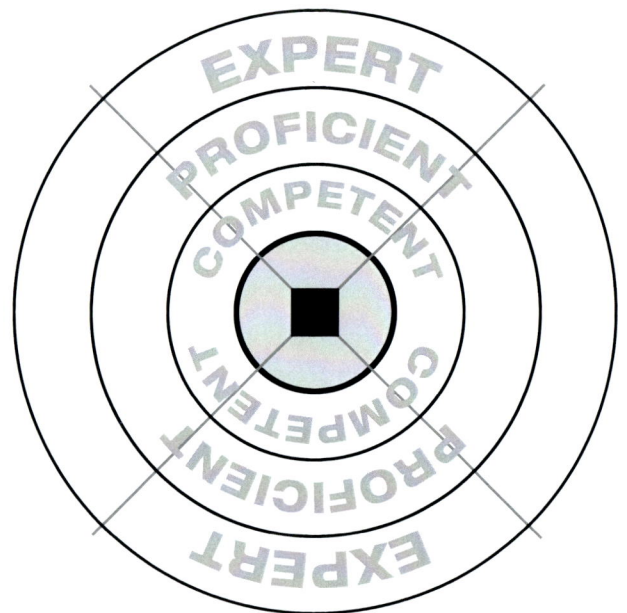

Statements indicative of performance levels can be identified and the levels recorded in diagrammatic form

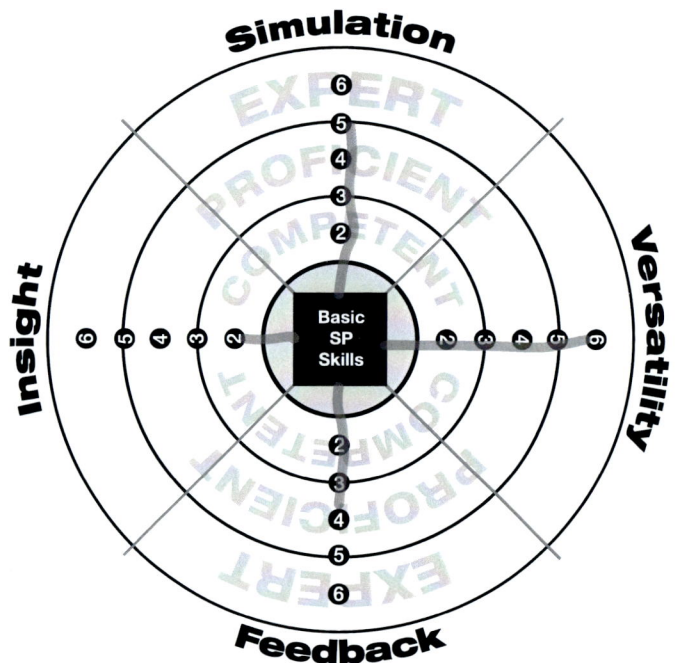

Expertise levels identified from indicative statements recorded as an episodic 'Fingerprint'

Domain: Simulation

Expert

- Can be relied upon for high-stake procedures
- Will absorb verbal scenarios and respond at the required level
- Responds authentically to bad news and other emotional upsets
- Realistically incorporates physical signs into scenario for examination
- Presents with different demeanours for multiple cases
- Simulates cases with complex medical and social history

Proficient

- Presents as relative, client or doctor with conviction
- Responds to learning purpose with understanding
- Simulates outline cases rapidly
- Responds imaginatively when required
- Is a reliable standardised patient for range of assessments
- Adds depth of character – expresses emotion realistically
- Responds uniquely in each consultation
- Original scenario/case represented consistently at each presentation
- Personal responses incorporated in role permanently
- Scenario/case personalised securely

Competent

- Sustains consistency as standardized patient
- Is treated as a credible patient
- Sustains mode of speech and body language throughout
- Is examined as requested
- Starts – stops – restarts – rewinds in role
- Minimally personalised
- True to scenario/case
- Incorporates history
- Checks clinical details (not caught out medically)

Basic SP Skills

Universal Principles

- Understanding the application of equal opportunities
- Observing confidentiality

Patient Case

- Learning the role
- Checking clinical behaviour
- Personalising the role

Learning Purpose

- Checking group learning level and purpose
- In action
- Responding in role – consistently
- Starting, stopping, winding back
- Being examined or providing a findings card
- Giving positive, level appropriate feedback in role

Developmental Themes

- Authenticity
- Consistency
- Individual interpersonal responses
- Standardisation

Domain: Insight

Expert

- Is sensitive to poor facilitation and knows why
- Gives feedback in appropriate learning language when asked to come out of role
- Knows when to come in and out of role credibly when self-facilitating
- Responds in a manner appropriate to case situation & purpose

Proficient

- Emotional reactions consistent with case character and approach of person consulting
- Sensitive to quality of facilitation
- Adds value to poor learning situation
- Introduces cues and clues responsively
- Increases or decreases response emphasis to match group or individual pressure
- Stays within simulated patient boundaries
- Responds to candidates in a timely manner

Competent

- Expresses feedback in a manner fit for group purpose
- Recognises the danger of reacting too personally to disapproved behaviour
- Avoids distracting detail
- Absorbs next move from listening to facilitator group discussion during 'time out'
- Fits group and/or facilitator purpose
- Enacts scenario/case in an audible and visual manner appropriate to the group
- Checks learning or assessment purpose
- Is aware of nature and learning level of group

Basic SP Skills

Universal Principles

- Understanding the application of equal opportunities
- Observing confidentiality

Patient Case

- Learning the role
- Checking clinical behaviour
- Personalising the role

Learning Purpose

- Checking group learning level and purpose

In action

- Responding in role – consistently
- Starting, stopping, winding back
- Being examined or providing a findings card
- Giving positive, level appropriate feedback in role

Developmental Themes

- Responding to learning needs while remaining true to the patient's or other voice
- Recognises group learning needs while enacting a scenario/case
- Response to situational requirement of case

Domain: Versatility

Expert

- Is self and another self when self-facilitating
- Switches case history, mood, demeanour convincingly as different SP in the same session
- Presents case convincingly in a variety professional situations
- Sits, speaks, responds in basic to complex roles appropriate to the professional situation

Proficient

- Incorporates physical signs beyond normal social demeanour
- Devises constructive ways to help inadequately facilitated group
- Individualises complex scenario/cases
- Demonstrates range and depth of response
- Responds creatively to unforeseen requests
- Nuances role to fit with facilitation
- Uses a range of communication skills as appropriate for the role

Competent

- Responds emotionally with care
- Communicates non-verbally
- Responds uniquely in each consultation
- Presents with matching demeanour and physical signs
- Presents with distinctive personalisation
- Makes subtle changes to dress

Basic SP Skills

Universal Principles

- Understanding the application of equal opportunities
- Observing confidentiality

Patient Case

- Learning the role
- Checking clinical behaviour
- Personalising the role

Learning Purpose

- Checking group learning level and purpose

In action

- Responding in role – consistently
- Starting, stopping, winding back
- Being examined or providing a findings card
- Giving positive, level appropriate feedback in role

Developmental Themes

- Range and quality of response in role
- Degree of differentiation in different scenario/cases
- Adaptation to facilitation

Domain: Feedback

Expert

- Touches upon personal issues acceptably
- Challenges constructively in feedback debate
- Will provide out of role advice with reluctance

Proficient

- Provides individualized personal feedback on request in role only
- Is observant and objective for summative+ evaluation
- Out of role feedback may use interpersonal skills language
- In-role employs non-specialist language to name interpersonal skills
- Feedback succinct and helpful, were possible for future behaviour
- Individual feedback neutral – avoiding damaging self-image

Competent

- Feedback given in consistent voice in everyday language
- Feedback descriptive not interpretive
- Feedback attuned to group learning purpose by faciltator
- Feedback unbiased, constructive and polite
- Feedback rules observed

Five feedback rules

- Check whether feedback required in or out of role – or both
- Focus on observed behaviour, not the person
- Focus on what is seen and felt
- Focus on description rather than judgement
- Focus on specific behaviours within the context in which they occur

Basic SP Skills

Universal Principles

- Understanding the application of equal opportunities
- Observing confidentiality

Patient Case

- Learning the role
- Checking clinical behaviour
- Personalising the role

Learning Purpose

- Checking group learning level and purpose

In action

- Responding in role – consistently
- Starting, stopping, winding back
- Being examined or providing a findings card
- Giving positive, level appropriate feedback in role

Developmental Themes

- Distinction between individually relevant and general feedback items

SP Expertise Example

SP-EBW - 'Being' Mrs Judith Anderson

Reason for the case

The patient consultation recorded for the role which became Mrs Judith Anderson, age 63, was thought to be sufficiently complex to challenge even the most experienced GP. Fourteen doctors were recorded consulting with Mrs Anderson in their own surgeries, and the films scrutinised independently as part of a research enquiry. The case was adopted by EBW and presented to doctors in such a way that the challenge remained consistent from doctor to doctor.

First impression

My first impression, when I saw the tape, was of a very complicated personality. She appeared to walk with some difficulty and to sit down very slowly. She was dressed smartly and her hair was neat. In her hand she was carrying what appeared to be a small cardboard packet. I thought she had a slight tremor but wasn't sure. The doctor welcomed her and she went on at great length about forgetting why she had made the appointment. As the doctor didn't interrupt, this was followed by a long account of her current symptoms. As I was of a similar age and felt an affinity with her, I agreed to take on the role and began the task of transcription. We are obliged by the Leicester method to write down exactly what we see and hear on the recording.

Absorbing the recorded case

The patient wanted to know what was wrong with her. She was in pain when she woke up in the morning and was having concentration problems. In addition, she had to sit down to come down the stairs. She had seen a specialist in outpatients but the several kinds of prescribed medication had distressing side-effects and made no difference to her symptoms. The GP said an occupational therapist might help and then asked why she was carrying a Nexium pill box. She replied,'Oh yes, that's why I've come. I want to reduce the dose'. Because of the doctor's willingness to listen, her story became more and more complicated. She told the doctor that if she were to have a serious stroke, she didn't want to be resuscitated. That was put in her notes and she signed it. She went on to say that her husband wouldn't listen to her.

A letter from the neurologist stated that while she had Parkinsonian symptoms, she had not responded well to any of his suggested treatments. He suspected she had multi-system atrophy.

Help with body language

A very experienced SP colleague was very helpful. We looked at the film together and practised how best to move and replicate the patient's body language, which helped to build up my confidence.

Checking with the originating doctor

I was ready with a long list of questions when I met the originating doctor. We watched the tape together and then did a trial consultation. The doctor asked the questions more or less as he'd done with the original patient, then he posed other questions to explore different corners of the case – this to prepare me for the range of questions a variety of doctors might ask. I tried to use the patient's language and was given helpful feedback

I learnt that the Nexium pill box she sat holding in the video was empty, and that these prescribed tablets were to protect her stomach from side-effects of other drugs. In the video, she said she'd taken her books back to the library because she 'Can't read any more'. This puzzled me but the doctor thought it was a concentration rather than an eyesight problem. I also learnt about her tremor. She was worried and anxious, maybe with some depression. What she really wanted to know was whether she has Alzeimer's or Parkinson's.

Family wise, I learnt she had two grown-up children who she rarely saw. More important, her husband treated her coldly and didn't engage with her problems.

Out on the road

The doctors I consulted with had read the notes and the letters before I was called in. Some chose to deal with various different parts of the problem. It was an awful lot to be landed with if you were meeting Mrs A for the first time! I was able to use the long introduction Mrs A used initially with many of the doctors I saw. I was also able to use some of her questions: 'Would a brain scan help? One of my friends was diagnosed with Parkinsons by this method.'

Using the Leicester method we know we must never add or elaborate on medical symptoms beyond the initial brief. So if asked about a symptom not discussed with the originating doctor, we say 'No I don't think so, or I haven't noticed' This avoids taking the doctor down the wrong path and it's a matter of being consistent. Whereas, with questions about their life world, we have to imagine what the patient might say and thereafter absorb the answers into the patient's narrative. From one consultation to the next I had to improvise as questions came up:

Would you like to go on holiday?
Yes, I would love to go on holiday.
Would you like to visit your children?
Of course, but they are both very busy.
Would you like to see a counsellor?
It would be great to have someone to talk to.
Do you think you might ever leave your husband?
Probably not, it would be an enormous step because I can't manage by myself as I need help with shopping and driving.

Comparison with the Edith Somers scenario

Most scenarios present cases in a similar manner to that of Edith Somers (Chapter 3) but Mrs Anderson was a completely different kind of task. With Edith there was a lot of personality help; she was a teacher so that rang all sorts of bells. With Judith Anderson, I could hear what she said, but what I read about her health problems was totally outside my experience. The purpose was also different: Edith was written as a means to practise medical history taking with groups of undergraduate medical students; Judith had private consultations with very experienced doctors observed only by the camera. For this there had to be total involvement and concentration in order to represent her faithfully in a unique and idiosyncratic consultation. With a scenario, there's much more leeway because you can personalise it and may repeat it with 'time out' interventions as directed by a facilitator. I had to 'be' Judith Anderson in mind and body until leaving the consulting room.
SP - EBW

Suggested Domain Statements Observed

Simulation

Expert

- Can be relied upon for high stake procedures
- Simulates cases with complex medical and social histories

Proficient

- Responds imaginatively when required
- Responds uniquely in each consultation
- Personal responses incorporated in role permanently

Insight

Expert

- Responds in a manner appropriate to case situation & purpose

Proficient

- Emotional reactions consistent with case character and approach of person consulting

Versatility

Expert

- Sits, speaks, responds in basic to complex roles appropriate to the professional situation

Proficient

- Incorporates physical signs beyond normal social demeanour
- Demonstrates range and depth of response

Feedback

Expert

- N/A

Proficient

- Provides individualised personal feedback, on request, in role only

Facilitator Expertise Development

Does group-work practice exemplify a wider societal value?

'All that remains essential for open societies is that there are rules of engagement which allow the continuation of the process of trial and error. The whole point of the open society is that there is not just one way, nor are there two, or even three, but an indefinite, unknown .. number'.

Ralf Darendorf, Karl Popper Lecture, LSE, (1989)

Facilitator behaviours can be recognised according to four activity domains

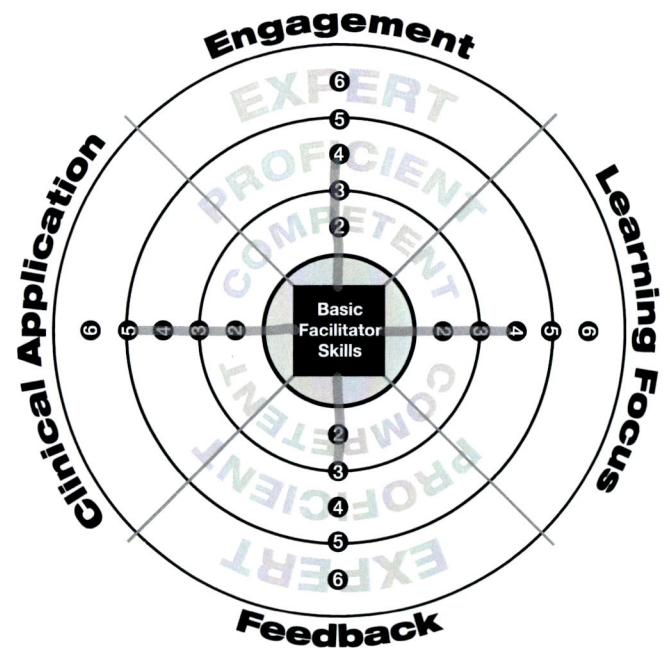

Expertise levels identified from indicative statements recorded as an episodic 'Fingerprint'

An important juxtaposition for SP facilitation? Are both feasible?

Behaviour theorists argue that deliberate practice, as facilitated by informed feedback, allows practitioners to minimize errors. Whereas, cognitive theorists suggest that improved performance results from practising complex tasks that produce errors – errors that provide rich feedback applicable to future performance.

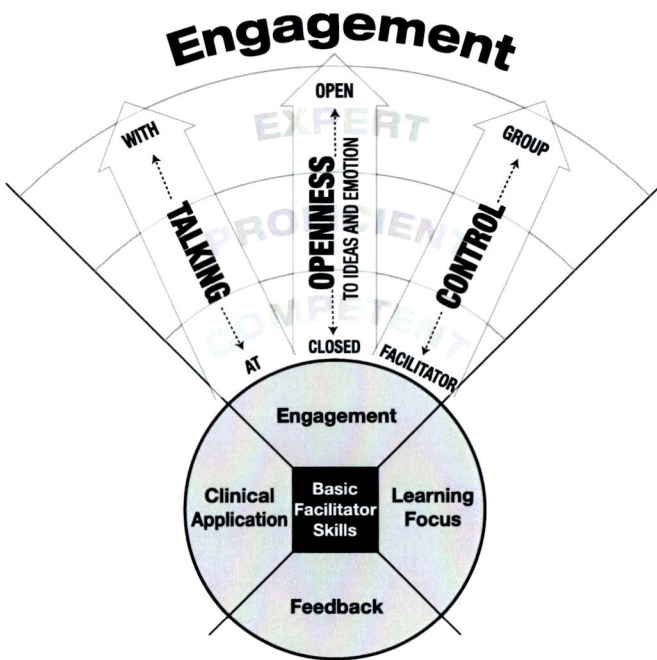

Facilitator Action Dimensions

Statements indicative of performance levels can be identified and the levels recorded in diagrammatic form

Domain: Engagement

Expert

- Group members bond with complex programme
- Content and process seamlessly linked to practice
- Criticism/dissent managed constructively
- Session timed to group agenda
- Takes individuals and group out of comfort zone
- Personal characteristics and values discussed constructively
- Shows awareness of bigger picture
- Facilitator direction accepted collegially
- Encourages mature group processes to flourish

Proficient

- Learning purpose explored collaboratively – agenda negotiated
- Participant distress resolved
- Different aspects of programme interact to good effect
- SP scenario/case used in reference to work based practice
- Facilitator interjection taken as point for discussion
- Encouragement of patient's feelings in discourse
- SP accepted as learning resource – alternative approaches explored
- Members interact across the group
- Facilitator models neutral chairing
- Group confidentiality assumed
- Timing negotiable
- Promotion of mature group processes in terms of trust, openness, robustness of challenge

Competent

- Session follows outlined structure with evidence of active learning
- Projected timing observed

- Some members feel free to talk about feelings
- There are examples of inter-group discussion
- Interaction appropriate to group size
- Group members contribute on request
- SP scenario treated as a personal test by group members
- Group follows facilitator guidance

Basic Facilitator Skills

Temperament

- Calm & Measured
- Non-directive

Universal Principles

- Understands application of equal-ops in groups
- Constantly works towards self and group determined learning

Clear processes

- Seating – Use of SP – Group tasks - Observation – Making mistakes – Trying new approaches – Feedback rules

In action

- Keeping time – Use of challenge – Switching control – Learning check

Developmental Themes

- Moving from directive to minimal direction
- Encouragement of inter-member collaboration
- Negotiating agenda control from facilitator to group
- Inclusion of emotional with cognitive responses

Domain: Learning - *Process*

Expert

- Group continues previous session topic – in-depth discussion
- Work-based practice and associated feelings exposed for colleague and facilitator comment
- Advanced use of interpersonal skills and behaviours identified
- Issues such as bereavement, terminal illness, psychiatric conditions, patient complaints, medical malpractice are approached sensitively through SP scenarios
- Integrates theory with observed practice
- Range of insights in play

Proficient

- SP scenario/case is treated holistically
- Group establishes a collective record of what is seen and heard
- Alternative experience sought as stimulus to personal learning
- SP case considered in relation to time used
- A range of interpersonal skills identified by observers
- Opportune learning items briefly integrated
- Clarifying motive and meaning of action between person consulting and SP comes from within group
- Requests to try alternative strategies are made – learning purpose adjusted

Competent

- Learning Capture techniques identify basic skills reinforced
- Observations are explored to establish meaning
- Sharing of experience encouraged
- Minimal opportunity is taken to try different tactics
- Most group observers record discrete behaviours
- What happens can be related to specific interpersonal skills

- Interaction driven by a declared learning framework
- Learning purpose is clear and SP used to support that outcome
- Group defers to the facilitator's declared learning purpose

Basic Facilitator Skills

Temperament

- Calm & Measured
- Non-directive

Universal Principles

- Understands application of equal-ops in groups
- Constantly works towards self and group determined learning

Clear processes

- Seating – Use of SP – Group tasks - Observation – Making mistakes – Trying new approaches – Feedback rules

In action

- Keeping time – Use of challenge – Switching control – Learning check

Developmental Themes

- Encouraging professional reflection
- Identification of clinical application
- Mutualising – learning from each other
- Supporting the necessity of individualised learning
- Making a habit of group members' search for meaning and alternative approaches

Domain: Clinical Applicaiton - *Content*

Expert

- Facilitator awareness of own attitudes and values
- Clarity about levels of competence; possible need for external help
- Indicates sources of relevant information and experience
- Elicits boundaries for action
- Helps sustain balance of patient-centredness v. doctor responsibility
- Assists with problem solving priorities

Complex Cases - e.g.

- Deeply emotional cases
- Complex psychiatric issues
- Complaints
- Complicated PMH + new problems
- Doctor appraiser training
- Refresher courses for senior staff

Proficient

- Clarifies transition from frameworks/ checklists to real life situations
- Understands members clinical context
- Identifies way to link patient-centredness with clinical safety
- Helps identify clinical uncertainty
- Elicits links between workplace experience and SP scenario

Standard Professional Cases - e.g.

- GP practice patients
- Training workshops
- Telephone consulting
- Concordant management
- Breaking bad news

Competent

- Uses frameworks and checklists
- Links cues to more secure diagnosis
- Concentrates on achieving a complete history

- Medical Training

Basic Facilitator Skills

Temperament

- Calm & Measured
- Non-directive

Universal Principles

- Understands application of equal-ops in groups
- Constantly works towards self and group determined learning

Clear processes

- Seating – Use of SP – Group tasks - Observation – Making mistakes – Trying new approaches – Feedback rules

In action

- Keeping time – Use of challenge – Switching control – Learning check

Developmental Themes

- Clinical – community health – interpersonal knowledge considered for safe practice
- Situational – work-based experience incorporated
- Identification and consideration of clinical uncertainty
- Practical implications of patient-centred approaches

Domain: Feedback

Expert

- End of session personal learning exchange may become a joint commitment to action
- Feedback prompts deep exploration of clinical and related interpersonal skill issues
- Discussion focused on matters concerned with group members' professional work
- Interaction at appropriate level for age and experience of the group
- Emphasis on encouraging all members to respond to items of feedback
- Emotional responses considered as important aspects of professional life
- Issues of self-image and denial confronted constructively
- Individual and group behaviours challenged opportunely

Proficient

- Group shares end of session learning
- Formulaic interaction recognised
- Distinction between exam techniques and future good practice acknowledged
- Interaction appropriate to professional level of group
- Emotion considered without potential distress
- Challenge to future professional behaviour incorporated into reflective discourse
- Feedback responses sensitive to individual learning styles
- Feedback omissions highlighted
- Feedback procedures introduced, revised if helpful and corrected if not followed
- Most group members contribute voluntarily

Competent

- There are signs of proficient behaviour
- Session-end learning feedback limited to session purpose
- All feedback given in role
- Alternative interpretations introduced
- What happens considered in terms of what, how, and why
- Most group members make constructive contribution when asked
- Discussion limited to agreed learning focus
- Feedback rules revised at commencement of session

Basic Facilitator Skills

Temperament

- Calm & Measured
- Non-directive

Universal Principles

- Understands application of equal-ops in groups
- Constantly works towards self and group determined learning

Clear processes

- Seating – Use of SP – Group tasks - Observation – Making mistakes – Trying new approaches – Feedback rules

In action

- Keeping time – Use of challenge – Switching control – Learning check

Developmental Themes

- The distinction between curriculum and professional purpose and assessment requirements is clear
- The power of SP action plus group feedback on future behaviour is manifest through skilled facilitation
- Adapting feedback rules according to group members' experience
- Relating feedback responses to learning purpose and consultation frameworks

Facilitator Expertise Example

Dr LF - Facilitating a Two-Day Course

The course

Sponsored by The Cancer Network, the course is open to those looking after patients with cancer and long term conditions, and there is also an end of life focus. Participants include hospice staff, senior hospital physicians, surgeons and nurses as well as community matrons and related staff. Sometimes there are chaplains, occupational therapists or dieticians.

Those attending often have substantial experience. The nurses are likely to be in the senior pay bands with at least five years' experience. The doctors will have ten or more years' experience and be consultants or in their final years of registrar training.

My task is to support everybody in developing and extending their communication skills, mainly through exploring situations that have challenged them.

Participant preparation

The workbook, which people receive before the course, should take several hours to complete. It reviews a wide range of professional opinion including: evidence supporting the importance of effective communication and personal reflection; the current national drivers; what the NHS requires and what patients want from health care professionals, particularly in terms of communication behaviours and values. For example, a patient may say, 'I want someone who is honest', or 'Someone who understands me', 'Someone who listens', or 'Someone who thinks of me as a person not just an illness'. This is both an attempt to prompt thinking about challenges related to these patient feelings and also to inspire confidence that the benefits of attending the course will be of value

The workbook asks people to think about a challenging situation they've had in which they feel communication was a key element. This might have been with a patient, a relative or with a colleague. It's common to hear people talking about meetings called to discuss a patient's cancer treatment, where they have to deal with an overbearing or difficult colleague. We try to consider all aspects of professional life, not just those that deal with patients. When they come to the course we set up a working agreement in order to enable safe disclosure; how best to deal with the personal challenges they've faced and the feelings they have about them. At this stage we need to get an idea of the range of examples. They might describe dealing with an angry or upset patient, or of being asked to collude in not telling a diagnosis, or dealing with people in denial.

Activity One – sharing communication experience

The initial sharing of experience not only highlights the generality of issues, it helps the group begin to feel comfortable. We then spend time thinking about core communication skills, a kind of refresher using DVD clips, we look at what facilitates or inhibits communication. Eliciting and reinforcing comments from the group, we go on to think about cues and how a consultation might be structured. Historically, more time is spent in medical training and in particular, in GP training, on consultation skills and structure. For some nurses it is very useful to be more explicit on the structure, for example, setting the scene, having introductions, gathering information, negotiating a plan and closing the consultation. Other elements can also emerge, such as rapport building.

This leads on to consideration of what's important to patients and the consequent need for consultants to include a psychological focus in their interviews. We review previous experience of role play and share the rules that will, hopefully, make open discussion safe and promote learning. Next we get people to explain the scenario they would like to practise. Mindful of the fact that we have one male and one female simulator arriving at lunchtime, we find out whether scenarios require a male or female patient, relative or colleague.

Activity Two – preparing the role-play

After lunch we split into two groups of five with a facilitator and a simulator. Each group picks up one of the communication challenges, for example, one doctor reported a really difficult situation where it quickly became necessary to give some bad news, at which point the patient got really angry, very upset, and the doctor didn't know what to do. We establish the background to give the simulator a deeper insight. What is the family situation? What was difficult about it when they got angry? There may be clinical issues to clarify. We search for the challenge that is to be reproduced in the role-play, i.e. a verbal scenario. This first happens in the group, followed by a briefing with the simulator and participant outside the group to explore any underlying concerns. Then the facilitator and simulator fine tune what should happen; how it should begin, for instance. The group then prepares to observe and record specific behaviours (not opinions) for feedback.

Activity Three – recording and feedback

The role play is started and recorded with a video camera. The action may continue until the participant stops it or gets stuck – the facilitator may also stop it. This may be as short as a minute or up to 10 minutes. A clip is watched and commented upon with positive feedback and offers of alternatives. We then use the option to start again or rewind to the challenging section. In the final ten minutes of the session we bring together what has been learnt by the participants and members of the group. Hopefully, if things have gone as planned, an example of a

strategy for dealing with an angry patient will have emerged: listening without interrupting; acknowledging the anger – to name but two techniques.

Each participant spends an hour and a half enacting the role-play. Observers are therefore obliged to concentrate on the action for six hours. It's quite intensive! Micro breaks become necessary. As facilitator, I have to gauge the levels of engagement, and at times do things to raise the energy level in the room; often covertly but sometimes overtly. Achieving the same level of meaning for each member over two days can be tricky.

Activity Four – unfinished business

The unfinished business session is there to address communication issues that have not been dealt with in the role plays. This may involve watching video clips with discussion of what's effective, or information-giving exercises where the clinical relevance can be explored by all of us. It's useful to use a range of activities at this point to maintain the energy of the group and hopefully, their learning.

General issues requiring facilitator skill

It is essential that facilitators will, with different styles, use the experience and skills of the group so it is not only learner-centred in terms of people bringing particular challenges from their professional life but also that new learning emerges from the experience, i.e. it is self-directed.

Furthermore, it is necessary to be there as a facilitator rather than an expert or a teacher. Though there has to be a sense of trust and respect when working with professional colleagues, you do need to be in control. I'm among professional colleagues but I don't see myself as a member of the group if I'm there to facilitate it. I'm there to work hard and enable their learning.

More personally

There's a lot of process to manage. The course manual describes one way to do this, but juggling what happens and managing feedback is very personal; it's all about knowing what you want to happen. I've now seen lots of scenarios, enough for me to know, usually, where things are going. But sometimes a group gets stuck and you find them valuing poor communication skills. Rather than saying, 'That doesn't work', they say the opposite in their bid to be kind. I find that challenging. Feedback from the simulator can be a powerful voice in cases like that. In a similar way, if I'm not sure what the communication challenge is, involving the simulator in the discussion can be helpful as it can 'unblock' the situation.

There are always group dynamic issues, and managing non-participation in a respectful way can be difficult. It can be disappointing when a member picks a scenario that is too easy. Sometimes I don't spot it soon enough to challenge them. If I do spot it there is a chance to reset the scenario. Making the patient angrier, for instance, may cause them to learn rather than just showcasing their communication skills to the group.

We are very dependent upon the skill of simulators who occasionally struggle to make the situation realistic. Then you are stuck at a key point in the communication challenge. It's quite a task when a 25 year old simulator is asked to play a pensioner. The best ones are able to bring something very different to different roles in the course of two days. Occasionally more theatrical skills are called for. Playing colleagues tends to be more difficult as briefing them on all the aspects of the role is impossible.

Course facilitator demands

To be accepted as a facilitator, the course first demands seventeen days of your time. Three are as a participant, three shadowing a course, three on a trainers' course, and two days further training – after which you can help on courses and then be assessed running a course. It's a big ask. It requires consistency and handling people who don't want to be there.

Example of Suggested Domain Statements Observed

Engagement

Expert

- Group members bond with complex programme
- Content and practice seamlessly linked to practice
- Criticism/dissent managed constructively

Proficient

- Learning purpose explored collaboratively – agenda negotiated
- Participant distress resolved
- Promotion of mature group processes in terms of trust, openness and robustness of challenge

Competent

- Projected timing observed

Learning

Expert

- Work-based practice and associated feelings exposed for colleague and facilitator comment
- Advanced use of interpersonal skills and behaviour identified
- Integrates theory with observed practice

Proficient

- Alternative experience sought as stimulus to personal learning
- Opportune learning items briefly integrated

Clinical Application

Expert

- Facilitator awareness of own attitude and values
- Elicits boundaries from action

Proficient

- Understands member's clinical context

Feedback

Expert

- Feedback prompts deep exploration of clinical and related interpersonal issues
- Issues of self-image and denial confronted constructively

Proficient

- Interaction appropriate to level of group
- Feedback procedures introduced, revised if helpful and corrected if not followed

Competent

- What happens considered in terms of what, how and why

How to Use the Facilitator and SP Domains

Regard the domains as an attempt to identify progressive behaviour. Feel free to amend or add indicative statements to suit purpose. The four domains are analytical – behaviours may appear in more than one domain

Using the domains to make an expertise fingerprint

- Choose one domain

- Reflect back to a session and check statements to identify what you did

- Statements you identify will normally be at competent or proficient levels, or both (expert levels relate to sessions demanding more exacting and specific expertise)
- Do other statements suggest what you might have done differently?

- Consider which level the statements indicate – if entirely at one level mark the midpoint – if at two levels mark the level dividing line

- Repeat the process for the other domains

- Draw line from the centre to the four points marked – similar to the diagrams below – you now have a fingerprint for the session *and that session only*

Advice

- Do not try to memorise the statements – they are there to be scanned for recognition

- Do not expect to cover all the statements at one level – some only apply to particular groups and learning purposes

- A beginner who has fulfilled the Basic Skills will start at number 1 on the fingerprint circle

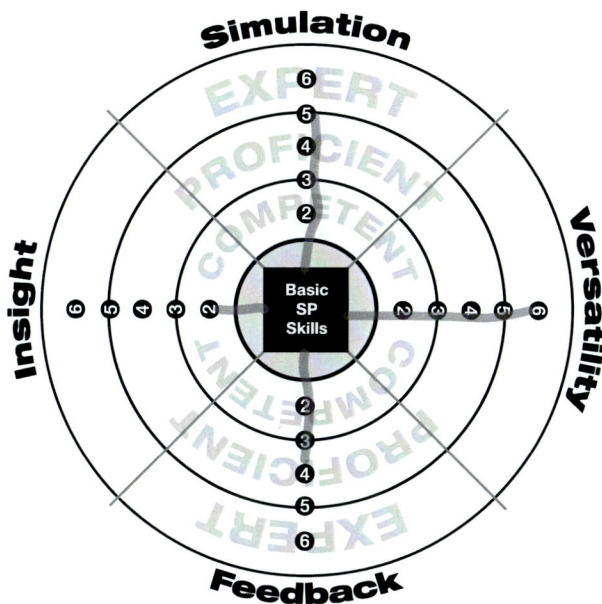

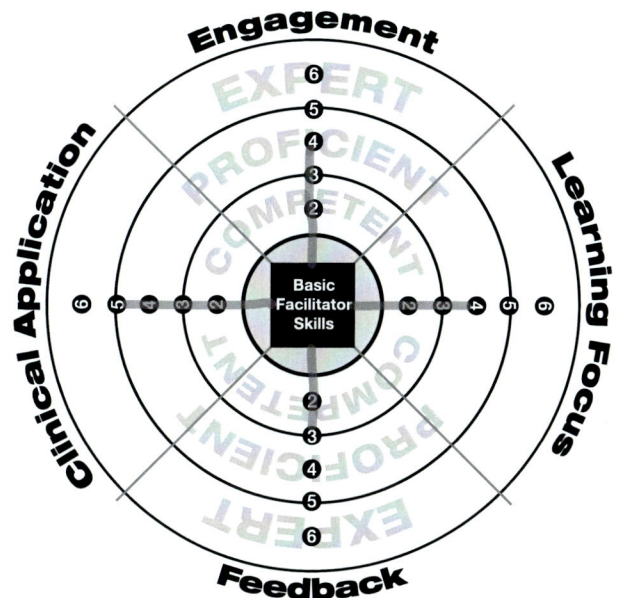

The domains should not be used for assessment. They are for formative use only

Chapter Eight

Opportunities

Looking back

The commitment to write *Light-Bulb Moments* and collect stories to illustrate the local range of SP usage was driven by my feeling that our East Midlands experience was being crowded out by high-tech simulation. This appeared to be compounded by lack of attention to the 'non-technical' or 'soft skills' we're normally concerned with. What I hadn't fully realised was a distinction between our way of working compared with other SP users at home and abroad. Travelling outside the region to conferences and courses has made me realise how differently other SP units function. All appear to be a result of local initiatives, with all the strengths and vulnerabilities associated with such origins.

In our experience the only nationwide control agency is the National Recruitment Office (NRO). They are concerned with the selection of GP speciality registrars for three-year training. The NRO needs to standardise the selection process across all UK regions. To that end, they demand the use of 'experienced' SPs and require specific training in the roles used for each succeeding year's selection centres – an impossible task without a cadre of reliable SPs.

Twenty years ago our initial group of four, supported financially by the then Deanery, now HEEM (Health Education East Midlands), grew to be a team of thirty plus, capable of providing a range of services backed up by the continuous experience of representing the patient voice in weekly workshops. Our training mode was the individual study of recorded consultations, with our character personalisation confirmed and clinical understanding extended by GP course organisers. Unlike SPs trained and supported for communication studies in medical school, and more particularly those trained for more

standardised provision as patient educators in well financed medical schools overseas, we had to be self-reliant. To a large extent this depended upon personal recommendation for inclusion in the team.

This manner of development is no longer feasible. Experienced members of the team grow older, and despite the problems of looking after our increasingly aged population, hardly anyone is writing roles for this age group (personal plea). Funding for non-technical training is minimal compared with the high cost of technical simulation, in comparison with which we are very low cost. More problematic is the regrettable fact that in our region there are little or no institutional drivers to develop or use SP services. This can be compared with the extensive use of a whole range of simulation 'modalities' in the Yorkshire and Humber Region.

Modalities refers to the ever increasing number of training opportunities offered by manikins, part-task trainers, digital technology and SPs, mostly focused on patient safety skills. However – and here the Yorkshire and Humber definition of clinical expertise involving patient communication can feed our optimism – there is a growing awareness that 'care and compassion' needs to be an integral feature of work across the simulation range. It is worth considering the view of an SP experienced doctor colleague that 'there will be no progress until health professionals learn to value the largely un-measurable soft skills'.

Looking forward

While reflecting on past experience and outlining a practical approach for self-reliant SP and facilitator skill development, I've concluded with suggested self-learner expertise domains; there for wider critique and amendment.

Our work with GPs, both trainees and practitioners, with its concentration on consulting skills, has led to in-depth consideration of interpersonal skills and their application in patient-centred healthcare. We know from experience how to use this language effectively for GPs. But, with appropriate adaptation, it can be used for integration in secondary care, mental health and community health training. These and associated group learning skills are transferable, with context specific help.

Meanwhile, in order to sustain authenticity our team needs support to ensure it can provide a service that reflects age, gender, and cultural diversity. This requires leadership from someone employed, probably part-time, to induct new people and ideally be sufficiently experienced to respond to new learning provision, impossible without regional or specifically commissioned support. We have been adopted and work under the imprimatur of the Trent Simulation and Clinical Skills Centre, for which we are very grateful. That is in the full knowledge that their resources are totally consumed by their own continuing programme needs.

The self-reliant approach – two strands of engagement

Over the years the team has been offering two booking strands:

- **Activity Strand One**
  An agency capable of providing SPs for a wide range of work, as witnessed by the stories in Part Two. Not mentioned so far is the supplying of SPs for interviews to identify consultants' person-to-person skills; assisting GP surgeries to establish a caring culture; regularly providing numbers of patients competent to prepare a role from an emailed scenario for the assessment of senior medical students' psychiatric skills; providing a range of SPs for CSA practice with ST3 GP registrars, and so on. Being able to respond to such requests requires a trusted, capable, self-reliant team. With such trust it is possible to respond to unpredictable requests. To do this with confidence, depends upon a quality of performance only achievable in our region with continuity of experience.

- **Activity Strand Two**
  Possibly the more locally idiosyncratic strand, and the most vulnerable, is the provision of SP directed workshops. Over the years such workshops have been designed and presented, with doctor help, to cover aspects of basic GP consulting and specific issues related to breaking bad news, telephone consulting, dealing with complaints, dealing with cultural diversity. We have previously provided SP surgeries for the assessment of GP consulting competence as well as surgeries to provide recorded evidence of allegedly incompetent GPs. More formatively, we have been able to present a range of recorded patient consultations for registrar physicians who were finding it difficult to achieve consultant status. This work strand saves doctor time, but requires SPs with specific knowledge of the health area covered.

To a large extent the first strand depends upon the experience gained from work in the second strand.

In the past much of this work was generated by word of mouth. Now there is a need for clever marketing, given the plethora of diversions within the current health world.

Opportunities – group learning with colleagues and SPs offers

Learning with SPs in a colleague group

Conditional on general learning factors

- Direct link with professional need
- Exposure of actual – real behaviours
- Integration of clinical or social need with interpersonal expertise
- Inescapable reflection on and in practice
- Focus on patient centred interaction
- Involvement of feelings
- Involvement beyond the comfort zone
- Engagement with a range from novice to expert participants
- Assumption of purpose designed for *quality* performance
- Can be custom built to local learning purposes

The opportunities for facilitated group work with SPs are many and varied, as are the opportunities to use SPs in non-group work, singly as in filming or collectively as for assessment procedures. Most medical schools already use SPs and have the financial and medical educators to design and promote sessions to fit their own curricula.

Suggested uses

Initial training

- Most medical schools use SPs for communication skill training. Indeed many SPs work across the undergraduate to postgraduate divide.

- I have little cross-region knowledge of initial nurse training. From asking around and reading it would appear that nurses have traditionally learnt their caring skills as an integral part of practical introduction to the skills required on a ward. Subsequently, these skills would be reinforced in-depth in the company of experienced mentors. Communication skills as a discrete element of training do not appear to have played a significant part. It seems this is unlikely to change given the volume of nurse trainees and cost of experienced SPs. Some nursing schools get round this by role-play.

- Some dental schools apparently use SPs for OSCEs. I have heard there is a particular need for volunteers with false teeth for training sessions. Plans are now in place to replicate the GP Selection Centre procedures for dentistry. This will require a cadre of experienced SPs.

Opportunities beyond current use appear to be slight in initial training

Secondary care opportunities

- Litigation and compensation costs hospitals a lamentable amount of money. Workshops concerned with methods for dealing with complaints using SPs could significantly reduce these costs as well as improving aspects of care.

- The 'health*care* achieved without compassion isn't healthcare at all' agenda has become highlighted in response to recent reports of malpractice and absence of care on hospital wards. Workshops designed for care and compassion learning using SPs could be a forerunner in this field. What is meant by 'mindfulness'? What cognitive constructs support the practical care skills? How do care and compassion inter-relate? Appropriate workshops could be scheduled for nurses, doctors and assistants as single sessions for different professional levels or integrated into the clinical work with low and high tech simulators.

- Trainers and facilitators using low and

high tech devices have to a large extent concentrated upon patient safety to the exclusion of 'soft skills'. There is now an opportunity to include interpersonal skills as an integral factor in these sessions;

- e.g. By combining a part-task epidural trainer with a simulated patient, the integration of communication and psychomotor aspects of the skill, such as the importance of patient positioning and dealing with discomfort while carrying out the practical procedure, can be rehearsed. Maran NJ, Glavin RJ, Low- to high-fidelity simulation – a continuum of medical education? Medical Education , 2003;37

- Managing patients with delirium and dementia in emergency departments is a particular example of a discrete area of cross-specialty hospital care that can benefit from an SP based training workshop attuned to a particular working context. There must be others.

Primary care

- There are group workshops in existence to help develop high quality consulting expertise for specialty GP training and remediation for those who continue to fail the CSA element of the MRCGP. There are a number of vocational training schemes within the region, most of which have used our services in the past. Servicing their needs requires new support provision.

- The existing *Refreshing Consultation Skills* workshop is well validated for post appraisal or revalidation support of GP practitioners. It needs promoting.

- Achieving consistency of practice in large surgeries can be promoted through whole practice sessions with SPs. This can have a profound effect but only if the session's interaction is sensitively planned with a level

of managerial honesty. Experience leads me to say, there are no quick fixes!

Integrated care

Providing SPs for a workshop with care workers in a home for patients with significant mental conditions is the only experience we have of working in the adult community care. If I understand it correctly there are three agencies providing services:

- Local Authority Adult Social Care providing direct care in the home and contracted out care home management to private sector companies

- Health and social care provision under the auspices of the local Clinical Commissioning Group (CCG)

- Partnership NHS Trusts providing adult mental health and disability support

Each of these organisations has well established practices to provide better community provision through a better alignment between Local Government and the NHS. The need for integration is driven by a variety of social, financial and political factors; providing better patient choice and freeing hospital beds, to name two of the most publicised. The integration of community care appears to be an arena of controversial change for some time to come.

As simulators we currently have no foothold in this community health field. Should this become possible, two areas of work seem worthy of consideration:

- At face-to-face levels care workers meet patients ranging from the disabled, elderly people in good health in sheltered accommodation to those with a variety of routine needs combined with time-to-time health and social dramas. Care workers ideally need to be trained to cope with those incidents that require personal initiative alongside routine responses to a whole range of patient conditions. **Work with SPs could be of inestimable value for the carers.**

- Those more senior people charged with integrating services, producing care paths involving a variety of agencies need to explore and practise new pathways along with training packages for new employees. **SPs could play an integral part in ensuring that the necessary skills are developed and embedded in future provision.**

Chapter Nine
Reflection

I started out by saying that our kind of person-to-person simulation is being crowded out by manikin-based and other 'high-tech' approaches, admittedly so crucial for clinical safety at a time when experienced trainers are diverted to front line service. Perhaps inadvertently, despite evidence that care and compassion has been lacking in some highly publicised cases, person-to-person care and compassion has become less of a training priority. This appears to be the case in our region.

I've recently been introduced to Julian Tudor Hart's Inverse Care Law:

'The availability of good medical care tends to vary inversely with the need for it in the population served. This inverse care law operates more completely where medical care is more exposed to market forces, and less so where such exposure is reduced'.

Hart JT, The Inverse Care Law. *Lancet* 1971, pp 405-12

I wonder if this reflects our current situation.

It's difficult to estimate the singularity of our East Midlands SP experience. SP involvement seems to be secure when integrated into recurrent training practice. Elsewhere it appears to be vulnerable. Nevertheless, we hope that opening up our stories and processes will prompt a wider dialogue. With dedicated sponsorship and a small financial support to assist the design of SP workshops, the approach illustrated here can be extended to assist group based learning for senior nurses, specific hospital needs and certainly, the future integration of community care provision – always basing such training around patient needs.

Protect the 'patient voice' in East-Midlands simulation

My intention was to explore simulation experience from a practitioner point of view. Not as a 'how to do it' manual, but as a text that can be dipped into as a means to develop expertise over time – a self-development approach. The expertise domains are included to provide 'dippers in' with confirmation of work done and suggestions as to what might be done differently. However, in thinking this through, I've become more aware of how dependent this approach is on continuity of experience, which in turn depends on stable support. That's always accepting that experience should ideally combine training and assessment episodes. Not forgetting that assessment requires a pre-determined patient response tailored to the assessment purpose; a specific form of SP expertise, in contrast to the singularity of the 'patient voice' required for most SP based training.

My initial emphasis was on the **range** of SP activity, as recounted in Part Two. I hadn't fully appreciated the implications of two distinct activity strands, one of which is more vulnerable than the other. SP experience is embedded in the medical school's curriculum. There are annual requirements for professional assessment. From time to time various health organisations choose to engage SPs for training and demonstration purposes or filming. The majority of Part Two stories exemplify this activity strand. Whereas, the *Telephone Consulting for GP Registrars and Refreshing Consultation Skills for GP Practitioners* workshops demand a different degree of SP engagement. These, and similar workshops are often presented by SPs who also self-facilitate small groups. Furthermore, it is vital that these SPs understand the nature of the training purpose.

That's why Leicester method roles are so important. They've enabled us to portray the 'patient voice' with some confidence – a unique resource for professional health training. And moreover, adopting these roles provides a form of training for the wider range of SP demands.

If SP work is to have a defining brand, it should be 'patient-centredness', enabled by SPs capable of presenting a near genuine 'patient voice'.

Understanding the learning potential of well facilitated SP group work is a key sub-text. Here again continuity is important for skill development.

We have recently prepared and presented a workshop on Patient-centred Consulting with the intention of achieving, at the very least, important professional insights.[5] All SP work is active by definition, usually related to workplace needs and acted out in the company of colleagues; conditions that create the likelihood for behavioural insight. It's worth adding a final point, that it's generally observation of colleagues that generates those spontaneous, and unpredictable, *light-bulb moments.*

[5] A description of a complementary workshop, 'Concordance focused practice: review of a simulated patient based workshop', can be found in Education for Primary Care, Vol 22, No 6, November 2011

Part Two
Case Stories

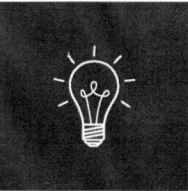

One _____

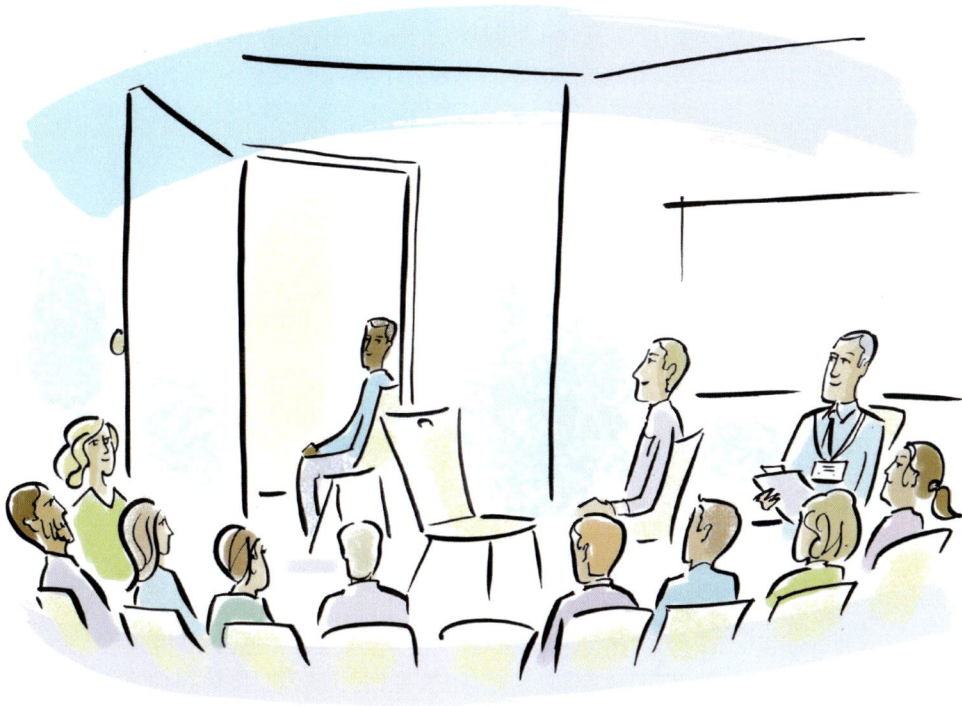

Simulated Patient Involvement in Consulting Skill Training

University of Leicester Medical School
Gary Aram

I started in general practice in 1980 and joined the General Practice Department at Leicester Medical School four years later. That's when my interest in simulated patients began. At the time, I knew of no one working in the same way but I quickly became aware of the potential for development. It was apparent that medical educators in America were far more practiced in simulation than we were. As I understood it, there was an assumption that UK patients would assist with teaching because the NHS provides free health care. That wasn't the case in America where they assumed fee-paying patients should not be required for teaching. As a consequence American medics already had 20 years of standardised patient expertise when I started weighing up what we should do here in Leicester.

First a bank of written scenarios

Colleagues and I at the medical school started to write roles with a view to accumulating a scenario bank with a wide selection of patient cases. These were based on written encapsulations of real patient consultations. I also felt it was important for fellow educators that the aims and objectives of each role and its key teaching areas were made explicit, be it history taking, examination, management, problem solving or relationships with patients. Somewhat later colleagues in the GP vocational training scheme derived their patient roles from video tapes of real patients and went on to use them for Simulated Patient Surgeries. However, we needed self-explanatory scenarios in order that SPs and facilitators would understand the challenges for each session – with a minimum of help! This required both a clinical and an educational approach!

Developing Simulated Patient Cases

We originally trained simulated patients using doctors – the doctor would have experienced a consultation, written a role relating to that consultation and trained the simulator. After the experience at Springfield Illinois, I decided patient integrity would best be maintained by training the simulator with a non-medical trainer. This should also improve the authenticity and presentation of the role, particularly if the trainer has SP development skills, which I don't believe all doctors have. So the trainer spec. was for someone with teacher experience, together with experience in the theatre and arts, who could develop SPs capable of portraying an authentic role that appears genuine to students. In doing this we avoided medical contamination within SP training. On completion of training, the role was checked by a doctor to ensure it remained authentic. By this process we improved the quality of our simulations.

The roles were written in a standardised format with the same headings and same criteria so that it was easy for a tutor to choose a suitable role. Indeed, we still use some of these scenarios. Happily, the format has stood the test of time with a little clinical updating here and there. Simulated patients were first used here in 1982. By 1994 we had around 18 simulators and a choice of more than 30 roles. Simulators were inducted into roles but weren't originally trained to give feedback. This was the next step I wanted to look at, along with the possibility of simulators becoming 'assessors' – one reason why I chose to check out what was happening in America.

Role Information Headings

- Character – Appearance
- Family & social backgrounds
- Work – Medical history
- Reasons for attending
- Expansion of symptoms
- Sensitivities areas – Management Reactions

Scaled-down version of detailed three-page SP Role information

John Edgar, age 55-60 is a reluctant attender who presents with physical symptoms of depression of which he is unaware.

He is not getting on with his wife, is stressed at work and resents his 21 year old son, who is off work because of stress and is at home all day. There are financial problems.

Howard Barrows unit at the University of Southern Illinois was impressive. They had a well-established belief that you can rely on trained standardised patients to assess student skills. The set-up is brilliant, a whole floor with individual consulting rooms all equipped with video connections to a central unit where you can see everything that's happening on monitor screens. The students go from one room to the next consulting with SPs who consult and assess independently *for assessment purposes.*

It was helpful to meet Howard Barrows. I came back with phenomenal enthusiasm. Though the restrictive factor was funding, I saw the OSCE (Objective Standard Clinical Examination) as a way to utilise this knowledge.

Devising an assessment process

It is no secret that assessment drives learning, but your assessment needs to be as close as possible to what you will be doing in practice – consulting, i.e. can you do the job? We were currently testing this with an essay question and a viva, neither of which proves you can consult: you might know the theory but can you translate that knowledge into appropriate behaviour in a medical interview with a real patient?

So we developed an assessment to be included in the end of session OSCE for Year I medical students – customarily a series of stations with different clinical or other course-based tests. However, you can't ask SPs to analyse problem solving; they soon lose their patient authenticity if they try! But they do have the ability to assess the content and manner of history taking, i.e. how might a patient be approached prior to a physical examination. What is the nature of any negotiation? Or, most importantly, will they return to see this doctor again? Will patients engage with the plan they've 'agreed' with the student? That's the proof in the pudding.

Another factor concerned the use of time limit within the OSCE. We wanted students to move away from taking a systematic routine history by following a checklist. This took a significant amount of time. We wanted students to pull out key information within a given time limit. To achieve that they had to actively problem solve; that's the important bit. The student must recognise: 'What do I need to know and how do I elicit it from the patient?' If you give them a time limit you can demonstrate more effective problem solving – you provide an opportunity for those students who are better problem solvers, to elicit the key information rather than going through a routine formulaic approach.

The assessment we designed incorporated a patient relationship fill-in sheet followed by a second sheet devoted to clinical problem-solving. In this we used models validated by the Howard Barrows Unit

Figure 1 Example of a Year One OSCE Observer/Patient Rating Scale

Interviewing and History taking	Achieved
Introduces self to patient	Yes - No
Puts patient at ease	
Allows patient to elaborate presenting problem fully	
Listens attentively	
Seeks clarification of words used by patient as appropriate	
Phrases questions simply and clearly	
Uses silence appropriately	
Recognises patient's verbal and non-verbal cues	
Exhibits well-organised approach to information gathering	
Behaviour and relationship with patient	
Maintains friendly but professional relationship with patient with due regard to the ethics of medical practice	
Conveys sensitivity to the needs of the patient	
Demonstrates an awareness that the patient's attitude to the student (and vice versa) affects levels of co-operation	
Overall Score	

It's very clear that there are key turning points within any diagnostic process. In the course, we emphasise that there are key negatives and key positives in any consultation. So, if you identify those key negatives and positives in a scenario, the simulator can tell you whether certain questions asked will trigger the appropriate responses. All the simulator then has to do is underline yes or no; did it happen in the consultation or not? So, because the clinical decision making is implicit in the questions on the evaluation sheet, the simulator is not making problem-solving decisions.

N.B. The below framework does not replicate teaching checklists/frameworks such as SQITARS or ICE. It's important that they start with open questions to let the patient tell his or her story. We encourage them to summarise what they have learnt with the help of the checklists to see whether they have covered all the appropriate areas. They have to listen, interpret and understand in order to repeat things back to the patient in a logical manner such as the patient can agree with.

Figure 2 Example of a Year One OSCE - Observational Clinical Framework

Identifies patient's reasons for consultation	Achieved
My wife made this appointment	Yes - No
I've been in bed for 3 – 4 days now	
I've felt like walking away from everything	
Considers physical, social and psychological factors as appropriate	
The pain is the same as before but worse	
The pains start 12 – 24 hours after activity and last for days	
I've been on the sick for 2 years now	
The doctors say my heart was fine and I have Costochondritis	
I take Naproxen 500mg twice daily	
My wife has had to stop work	
My son has stress problems and lives at home	
2 years ago there was a management change at work	
My wife and I don't get on like we used to	
Overall Score	

The simulator element in the course develops

The Year 1 course initially included three communication-skills sessions, each with a simulated patient case, originally limited to eliciting the patient's story; the history taking. We've now moved on to include management and information giving. During the pre-clinical years, students' main contact with clinical work is with simulated patients in addition to 'people and disease' visits, whereby the students develop relationships with two patients at home or in hospital. Year 3 becomes the clinical year at the end of which they do an Intermediate Professional examination (IPE). These assessments involve stations with simulators and examiners; for example, the student will have to explain to the patient why he is breathless after a heart attack. The patient will be primed to ask clarifying questions according to the nature of the student's explanation while the examiner observes clinical accuracy. The examiner confers with the patient regarding the manner and effectiveness of the interaction at the end of the timed session.

Originally we would only observe Year 1 OSCE consultations randomly in order to ensure reliability. Since then we've been obliged to change this by providing medical observers for each communication-based patient role because of the increasing possibility of legal challenge to non-medical markers. As a consequence, simulators no longer fill in the problem solving clinical check list, as before.

Simulators also adopt roles for the psychiatry assessment, and have recently been incorporated in the admission procedures for new students.

LAP provides material content and structure

The above story cannot be considered complete without mentioning LAP – the Leicester Assessment Package, elements of which impact on everything we do. Conveniently for us LAP was devised by colleagues in the Department of General Practice who did all the early research. LAP provides a detailed list of the strategies required to achieve consultation competence in five domains: history taking – examination – patient management – problem solving – relationship with patients. LAP has therefore provided us with a research validated framework from which we can choose both teaching and feedback items. The full scheme contains strategy lists more suitable for practitioners, from which we have selected items appropriate for various undergraduate course levels. For example, our history taking list for first year students is very practical:

- Introduces self to patient
- Puts the patient at ease
- Enables the patient to elaborate presenting problem fully
- Listens attentively
- Seeks clarification of words used by the patient as appropriate
- Phrases questions simply and clearly
- Uses silence appropriately
- Recognises the patient's verbal and non-verbal cues
- Identifies the patient's ideas, concerns and expectations (ICE)
- Considers physical, social and psychological factors as appropriate

All these items can be identified, practised and discussed during and after a history taking interaction with a simulated patient. They also provide the context for SPs to give constructive feedback in their own language, e.g. 'I felt comfortable talking with you' = puts the patient at ease. Simulated patients can easily use this language for scoring students.

We have been fortunate to have the authors of LAP as colleagues. Doubly fortunate because the LAP language we use and the consulting behaviour we try to develop by obtaining the patient's story, checking it and reaching a shared understanding, is entirely consistent with the 'patient-centred consulting' and 'holism' advocated by the Royal College of General Practitioners (RCGP).

To summarise: we chose to work with simulated patients to practise what happens in real life between doctor and patient. To do this well, we wrote detailed case scenarios based on real patient stories that include key aims and objectives for consultation-skill practice in small groups. Subsequently, we used the same or similar scenarios for OSCE assessments marked by the simulators. We later began to involve the more experienced simulators as agents in the learning process, about which more detail after considering the key to all this course development – the authenticity of the patient simulator!

The simulators

My concern with any new simulator is hidden agendas. We need to make sure they have no gripes about doctors, see whether their personal medical experience will interfere with any of the roles; for example, a recent bereavement. Nor do we want anyone who is going to be contaminated with prior knowledge, i.e. no medically trained personnel. Nor do we want people who will put on a performance – we have had worrying comments such as 'No problem, I've played all the major Shakespearian roles'. We've never advertised. Our simulators have all come by personal recommendation.

Most of them can portray a role. Some can do several roles distinctively. Once they have been trained to do the role the question is, how good are they at feedback? We've spent a lot of time on feedback training! So there are skill stages for SPs, 'I have a role', 'I can give feedback', 'I have been aware of contributing to an educational issue while in role because of the facilitator's feedback'. Patient based education is a better phrase –

giving a patient perspective. The *patient voice* has been increasingly recognised as being significant for patient satisfaction questionnaires, which are now so important for revalidation.

Having thought themselves into the scenario and *become* a recognisable patient, simulators have to be capable of cleansing and avoiding contamination. Contamination is about changing the role as a consequence of previous experience. Cleansing is about starting again without contamination. That said, as a facilitator I require some cleansing to start and stop *during* a learning session. Let's say the case management didn't go very well, so let's call 'time out', get the simulator out of the room and start again with a different student, but *winding back* to the start of management. To do this the simulator has to return and continue from the 'time out' moment (often repeating the last phrase used in order to help with continuity). When SPs are inducted into a new scenario it's important that there is sensitivity to cues. Cues are there to be picked up, so simulators need to understand the level of emphasis to apply if they are not picked up. Once the training is completed the role becomes standardised. Though the simulator will respond uniquely to different students, as in real life, the clinical elements of the role will be predictable and unchanging – unless of course they have to be adapted because of a change in medical practice.

The facilitators

New educators must have training to run a simulated patient session, and it is likely to be the hardest teaching they do. It's relatively easy to be a didactic teacher and go through set presentations. Teaching to a video is not too difficult, for example. Even student case presentations are manageable. But a simulated session can be different every single time you do it, potentially because there are different people involved. You have to think on your feet. The educator needs good analytical skills to recognise what is happening and relate that back to LAP. They need a good knowledge framework on which to hang what they are observing. 'Can I recognise what is happening in terms of the terminology?' 'Are the cues being picked up and responded to appropriately? Are the students using the triple diagnosis – eliciting Ideas-Concerns-Expectations (ICE)?' Facilitators need to know the LAP checklist and not just rely on their own clinical experience. The other dimension is engaging with the group, involving the simulator as a colleague (allowing time for them to give feedback), using the feedback process, arranging the chairs – I could go on!

Simulator educators

From the start, I was aware of simulators being used to teach students communication skills. Meanwhile, as a consequence of the feedback training, we became aware of the growing expertise of our SPs. Coincidently, we felt that our next step with the students was to create an opportunity for them to consult with SPs without facilitator direction. The bonus for this, and what sold it within the department, was that it would free up tutors to do other tasks. So we embarked on a trial run.

Initially, the tutor would introduce the session, ensuring the consultation was documented on the whiteboard according to a framework representing the hypothetico-deductive model, and that the students appreciated the necessary group processes: appointing a leader, use of time, computer access, having a break in the three hour session, for example. It is important that the group understands the need to create time to check the decision making evidence and plan the management. When the tutor returns to debrief, a summary of the clinical journey taken should be clear from the whiteboard – the group-appointed scribe having been instructed to 'minute' moment-to-moment decisions which can then be crossed out but not erased, as the differential-decision-making proceeds.

The simulator was required to maintain a role and give feedback throughout the process, but always in role until the debriefing, by which time he or she would have written a LAP format report on the whole session. An SP feedback example at debriefing might be; 'When the patient left the consultation he would not have followed the group's advice', followed by reasons why that would have been the case.

Students continue to give very, very positive feedback in their end of course documentation. They obviously enjoy the opportunity to work without tutor interference. They frequently comment that they feel liberated to try different approaches when unobserved. During the two hour period with the SP they can take breaks, delegate tasks to a group member, use books, access the internet and, of course, gain experience of collaborative working. Nowadays we don't even use a tutor to introduce the session; it's up to the group and the SP. The key for tutors is the clearly documented entries on the whiteboard from which they can analyse the problem solving.

Simulator educator sessions from an SP point of view

The way in which we conduct sessions is now detailed in the paperwork that underpins simulator-educator training workshops. It's a process that's been refined over time.

So, I have a clear procedure to introduce the session with students: I remind them about having a scribe, use of the whiteboard, not rubbing anything out, deciding whether to have a group leader or not, getting wide participation, asking for individual feedback for each of the three to four who will consult with me, using the internet/books to access information, having a break and so on. When we have finished that, I leave the room to get into character, from which point they know I will remain in role until the final part of the session when the clinical tutor arrives approximately 2.5 hours later.

Having such a clear framework leaves me free to be aware of what is going on in the group. Staying in character and not helping at all can sometimes be frustrating if the group is going miles off in the wrong direction; or someone is dominating the action or they forget to request feedback after they have taken a turn consulting (therefore making it more difficult for me to remember what I want to say, as I have to wait till the end). Sometimes, the students forget to ask for feedback because they're so intent on reaching the correct diagnosis.

I do enjoy watching the interaction between different students in the group – it's always different and I believe the students get a lot out of this process.

Staying in role for a long-time can lead to the odd glitch, such as occasionally realising you are responding in the third person, or worse, as yourself. Luckily, my current role is not that dissimilar to my own personality, so the students probably don't notice. I can imagine that a role where the character is very depressed and gives little eye-contact, would be much more difficult particularly for giving feedback. However, for those types of roles, we have been advised to 'lift' the depression a little for feedback, so still giving the feel of the character without all of the depressive symptoms. The 'examination' stage is a little tricky too, as the student isn't actually examining you, but just asking what the results would be if they examined you, and we read the answers off a card. As no patient would do this... it does spoil the illusion somewhat, but the students seem to have accepted this in previous Clinical Methods sessions.

I feel that students like the freedom to work in this way, which considering the double challenge of clinical problem solving in a self-organising group, leaves me feeling good.

We are not always needed to stay for the very final stage, where the tutor goes over the whiteboard with the group (going through what they have done, or what they perhaps missed or spent too much time on). I enjoy this part, and in my opinion it's nicer to stay and see it all through to the end. SP – DM

Dr Gary Aram was Senior Clinical Educator at the Department of Medical and Social Care, University of Leicester and is a practicing GP

Two

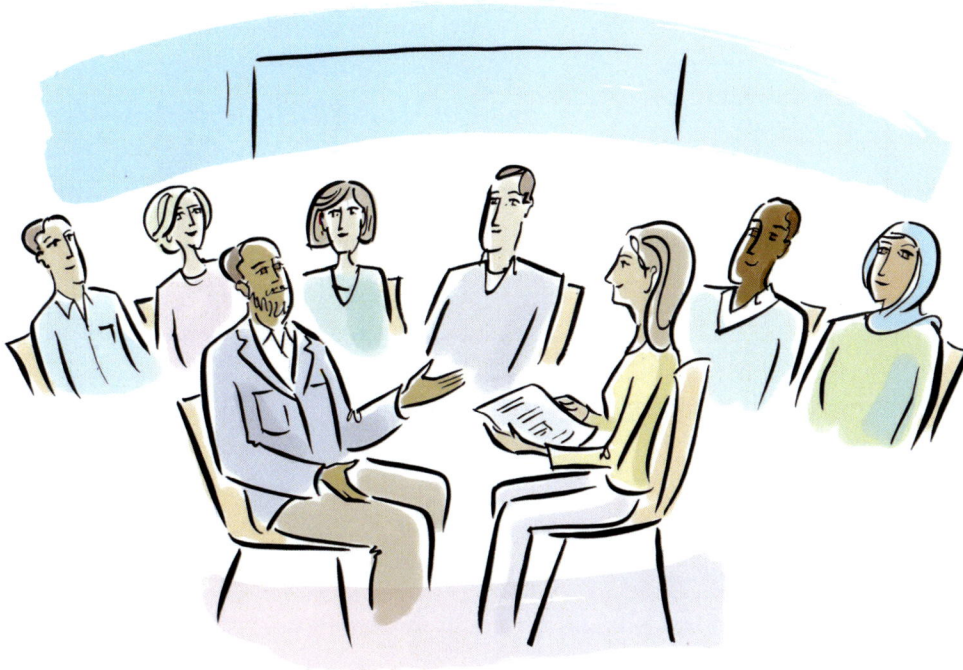

GEM School

(University of Nottingham – School of Graduate Entry Medicine & Health)

Simulated Patient Involvement in Module One Evidence Based Clinical Skills
John Frain

Context

The GEM School is attached to the new Royal Derby Hospital. We attract students from a mixture of graduate backgrounds many of whom have experience of health care settings – graduate nurses or pharmacists, for example. The vast majority will have done work placements. Whether they have experience of patient communication or not, we assume everybody starts at the same level. By the end of the first two years we need to make sure they can take a problem orientated history. They learn this in a modular fashion, so at the moment, they are concerned with the cardiovascular (CV) system. There are clinical skills which involve CV history taking and **at the same time** we try to teach formal interviewing skills which the evidence suggests are the most useful.

Student Learning Environment

The GEM school building has been designed for self-directed, team learning ideal for graduate students. Each group of 6 to 7 students has a team room with computer facilities. For each course module there is a *Workshop Booklet*. So students *can* arrive for each SP session with prior knowledge of Calgary-Cambridge and ALOBA action sequences. For some interpersonal skills they also have prior access to DVDs. Graduate students thus have a more mature learning environment suitable for the shorter degree course.

Course Evolution

Over ten years we have been on a learning curve ourselves. For instance, in the first couple of years we used to write scenarios and give them to the students in their small groups. One of the students, or sometimes a facilitator, would then play the role of patient in order that group members could, over time, practise taking a history. That was a very primitive way of doing it because:

(a)   we weren't really teaching communication skills and

(b)   the history taking was very much of a yes/no type of question and answer.

After five years our then Director introduced the Leicester simulators. That took a while to bed down but made an enormous difference in that we were also able to concentrate on the process of communication. The other thing we did near the beginning was to adopt the Cambridge-Calgary model for medical interviewing. We struggled with this content-v-process problem, more so because this is an intense course. We only have 18 months pre-clinical time. At the moment it's all organised on the basis of 9 modules, each of which lasts about 6 weeks. Each module comprises one or two communication and history taking sessions – one with the simulators and the other with real patients. The challenge has always been to teach the clinical content while, at the same time, teaching the skills to interview in a medical setting. Certainly, our students should be able to go onto the wards and take a history.

 By having a short presentation at the beginning of a session – say 20 minutes on cardio-vascular symptoms – we found students emphasised the content more than the process. So we shifted the presentation to the end of the session. Now they come to the simulation and practise their communication skills followed by a short whole-group session telling them what it all means clinically.

As a consequence, we now have two parallel sessions. The first, we call 'exploring symptoms', where we give the students written case descriptions for doctor-patient role play. Each case is orientated round a particular symptom. In the CV system there are 4 key symptoms: chest pain, shortness of breath, palpitations and swelling. All CV diseases come down to a combination of varying amounts of these 4 symptoms. So the students do the contents separately from the communication skills.

In the second session, we work on communication skills with the simulators. We begin with a 5 to 10 minute presentation to the whole group which might involve a short video showing them how the skill works in practice – by the time we've got to closed questions we'll have a short video showing how we would use the skills after taking a history using open questions, and after taking an opening statement. Following the presentation they now spend 40 minutes with each of four simulated cases thus leaving enough time for feedback. My feeling is that this works best. There is clear evidence of communication understanding and an equally clear link to the skill of the day. With each case, at least one person gets to conduct an interview at length and we can use the ALOBA framework to give highly structured feedback.

ALOBA: Agenda-Led Outcome-Based Analysis

ALOBA also provides a sequenced process for medical interviewing with SPs. For example, it starts with *Set the scene for the experiential work,* followed by, *Identifying the learner's initial agenda*, and concludes with *Closing the session*. Each of the 10 stages have elaboration suggestions.

Whether in the room for the introduction or for feedback and conclusion, experienced SPs will appreciate and be able to respond according to the ALOBA context.

SPs and the Learning Purpose

The module booklets and the SP role descriptions provide an explicit link to both the process and content. As an example we can compare statements in the Module One booklet and instructions in the SP briefing:

1. To practise communication skills

2. To gather the content of the patient's history

3. To attend to verbal and non-verbal cues

4. To receive feedback on your interviewing technique

5. To contextualise the patient's biomedical presentation within its psycho-social setting

Similar details in the Module Seven booklet will cover talking about emotional issues such as sexual history and using more advanced skills like sign-posting and signalling. These kinds of skills are mapped out over the 18 months.

Learning Purpose – SP Briefing for Sid Perry

- Develop the use of ALOBA
- Consolidate use of the following skills – Introduction – Taking an opening statement – Identifying an agenda – Using open questions to gather information
- Introduce the following skills – Use of closed questions to rule in and rule out further lines of enquiry
- Practise the following skills – Active listening – Summarising – Closure – Presentation
- Use of clinical reasoning to formulate diagnostic ideas

The learning purpose provides SP, Sid Perry, with direction for his feedback.

Sid Perry, 65 years

Biomedical perspective

My ankles are swelling up. It's been for a few years. We went on a coach trip last week and my feet got so swollen I couldn't put my shoes on. They used to go down overnight and come back during the day; now they never go down even if I wear those white stockings. My legs feel tight and painful. It's more difficult to walk. If I cut my leg water leaks out instead of blood. I had an ulcer on my leg last year and it took ages to heal. This week they've been particularly bad. I've been sitting around the house more as my breathing has been a bit bad. Now my legs seem really tense, red and shiny – worse than ever in fact.

Associated symptoms

Sometimes I feel breathless more than usual and my inhalers don't seem to work. I feel tired all the time. No weight loss – it's going up in fact – and no change in appetite. Started sleeping on two pillows instead of one. No chest pain, wheeze or temperature.

It's worth reinforcing the fact that clinical learning in these SP sessions is secondary to talking with the patient. That said the clinical briefing for Sid Perry is sufficiently detailed and authentic to be suitable for detailed history taking.

The 3 kids all live away

There's Edna's arthritis

What's all this about?

I've cut down on the fags, used to be 40 a day. Won't give up my beer. 2-3 pints a night and a 'few more' on the weekend

I feel a lot of discomfort. I have to use two pillows now instead of one and feel breathless. At least I haven't got any chest pain, temperature or wheezing.

MALE	SUMMARY OF TREATMENT CARD
Surname: Perry	Forename(s): Sid
Occupation:	Retired bus driver
N.H.S. Number	Date of Birth: Age 65 yrs
Date	Clinical Notes
Now	Legs: tight and painful, tense, red & shiny Difficulty Walking
1 year ago	Leg swelling down overnight Ulcer on Leg Well during the day
3 years ago	Swollen ankles and feet – can't put shoes on
40 years ago	Duodenal ulcer (vagotomy – pyloroplasty)
55 years ago	TB – isolation in hospital
Current medication	Flurosemide (2x daily)
	Smoker: 20 cigs p/day Drink: 50+ units p/week

ICEE

IDEAS
It's circulation, isn't it?
Bad breathing.... can be blood clots.

CONCERNS
I feel breathless; inhalers don't work.
Water tablets make swelling worse?
does this mean bad heart...kidneys?
Uncle Ernie had his leg off after his ulcer.
It's spreading up my leg.

EXPECTATIONS
I'd like treatment to drain off the water.

EFFECT
It's impossible to find shoes to fit.
My legs are restless and painful.
I used to enjoy walking,
now I can't.

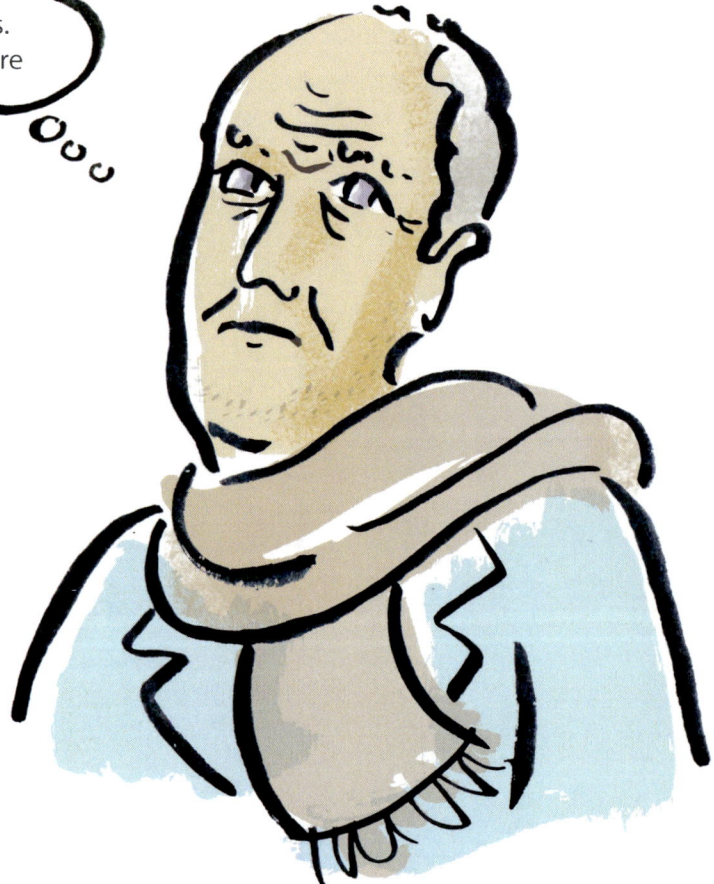

The Sid Perry case is complicated enough to fit our Module One purpose: **to concentrate on the patient and his symptoms, leaving clinical problem solving until later.** It highlights the interpersonal skills you need to achieve this and enable the maturity of our students to shine through.

Later on, we ask 'How would you like the simulator to play it?' More emotionally or tight-lipped, for example. There is a sexual history case which can be played in a variety of ways – one quite aloof and another guilt-ridden and emotional – and although they use the same words, the way it's done is transformed.

Facilitation

The facilitator, who may be a nurse, physiotherapist or doctor, establishes the chosen agenda and desired outcomes before distributing observer tasks and asking the consultant to bring in the patient. Depending on how much time is allowed for history taking and feedback in the 40 minute slot, another approach may be tried by a different group member.

Feedback follows the ALOBA sequence from a post consultation point of view with comments from the observers and the patient in role.

The groups then move round so the facilitator and simulator remain as a pair.

Four out of the six of us currently teaching the course have been to Cambridge to observe student teaching and do the communication skills course run by Jonathan Silverman. So we're trying to teach as we've been taught. We also work with the local NHS clinical skills team who've had similar training. Some of our facilitators are not GPs but are working in clinical skills in the Trust. Incidentally, they increasingly include communication skills in some of the scenarios they do with more senior students and doctors. Every summer we discuss what we are doing in the light of student feedback. We also run a simulated session to try out what we plan to do next.

Outcomes

One of the challenges for any communication skills course – a GP area of special interest – is what happens when they get onto the wards. They may not see senior or junior doctors communicating with patients in the way we have tried to teach them. I've had this conversation with Jonathan Silverman: it's all very well trying to teach them these skills but if they are not role-modelled when they get onto the ward – particularly in some specialities, no disrespect – they catch the idea that a surgeon is very definite and doesn't take any nonsense and some people will see that as the way to go.

Given the mix of students' past experience, Module One has always been a bit sticky. There are some students who've worked in our way before; some are perfect communicators and cannot be taught anything, and there are others who are OK with it. This year we didn't get any feedback of that kind, so I'm hoping it represents a sea change, in the sense that our skills are now so good we can get it across. In the last couple of years we've introduced the SPs earlier. We now have a session called 'The Opening Statement' which we do in the first weeks before they go out on their first GP visit. It's about inviting the patient to start talking and it fits their capability. That's gone down well.

Feedback on our use of SPs has always been very good. There have been disagreements on how we actually use them and how we construct the sessions but, in terms of sitting down with a patient and trying to interview them, students always find that positive and authentic. The scenarios are now more detailed, providing a wealth of material, and we've given more time to deal with them. Overall at the end of the 18 months they are very comfortable and can see the point of it.

SP reflection

What makes me smile when I go to GEM is that students maybe feel they can't do it, then do it without realising. I often praise them for the conversational moments when I feedback in role. 'It felt like it was a flow and I felt you were right there with me because of what you were saying about … '. It proves that communication skills are conversation skills – human skills. It's not medical skills!

You don't have to be a doctor to do a good history – I could do a good history, it's human interaction skills. SP - RMP

Dr John Frain is Director of Clinical Skills at University of Nottingham School of Graduate Entry Medicine & Health and a practicing GP

Three

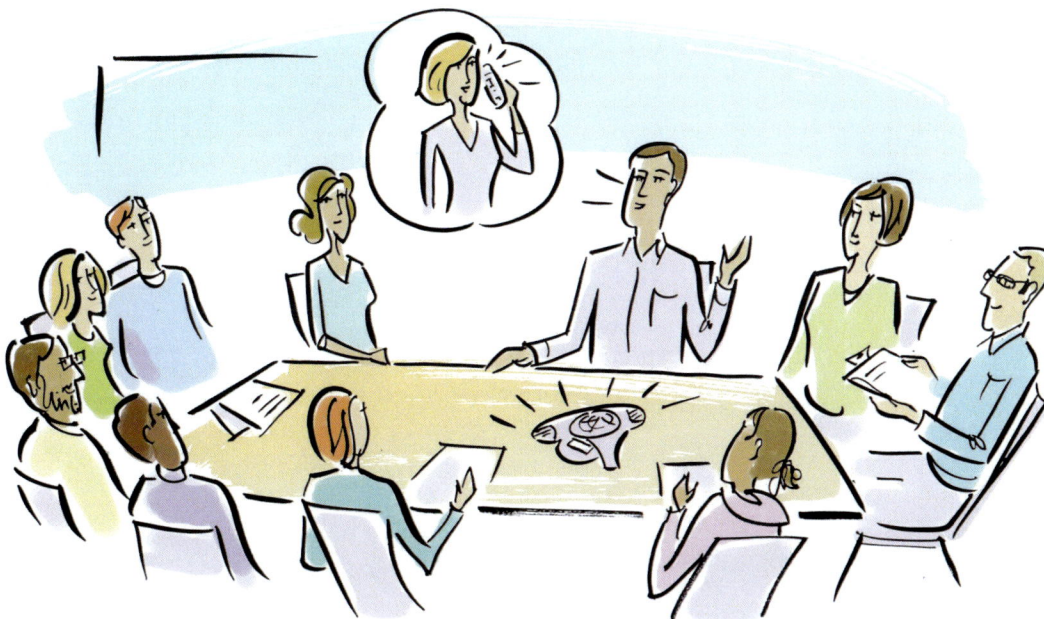

Telephone Consultation Workshop for GPs

Megan Murray

Origins

The Telephone Consultation Workshop is a three-hour session for GP speciality registrars. It was created collaboratively by GP course organisers (now programme directors) and SPs. From the start there was an assumption that it would be SP facilitated with an experienced GP in attendance to add features of clinical reality. Although out-of-hours triage and NHS Direct already provided assistance on the telephone, this workshop was prompted by the introduction of telephone consultations to alleviate Monday morning demand on already busy practices.

The focus is on high quality consulting, and offers ten registrars the opportunity to work with a 'distant patient'. Because the telephone used has a conference facility, each member of the listening group can give feedback. Group members are allocated a specific observational task. Though the 'distant patients' are out of sight in another room, they are close enough to slip their rapidly written feedback under the door for the doctor on the telephone. The sequence of patient roles is constructed to cover vital skills required for safe consulting. In order to limit costs, three SPs each cover three or more roles during the session.

To offer maximum impact SPs are required to adjust their voice tone and over-the-phone characteristics to match three or more cases convincingly.

On reflection, it is clear that this type of workshop requires continuity with GPs to keep content up to date, and continuity of SP team membership to enable the process to work smoothly. This is particularly the case with telephone consulting as there is no direct contact with the facilitator during the session.

Telephone Consultation Workshop

Programme

SETTING – Seating for 10 participants with SP facilitator & experienced GP, around one large table with conference facility telephone to ring up to 10 'distant patients' in another room

INTRODUCTION – Difference between face-to-face and telephone consulting – discussion of previous experience and perceived issues

HANDOUT – Summary of workshop key-points for reference throughout session

ACTION – Sequence of telephone consultations with some observers recording details of telephone specific skills and others recording the interpersonal skills used, followed by feedback after each patient. Patients provide written feedback

WASH-UP – Completion of Learning Capture Sheet with outline personal checklist + cross group exchange

Example of telephone scenario given to SP (for personalisation)

Origin of call

In surgery hours	✓	Out of hours	✗
On-call	✗	Inter-professional	✗

Patient	Dennis Ruskin
Age	70
Status	Retired quantity surveyor
Home circumstances	Carer for wife age 69 with MS and wheelchair-bound
Time of Call	3.30pm
Reason for Call	You have fallen and hurt your arm badly and do not know whether it is broken (it isn't)

Patient Information

Physical

- Fallen on left arm (right handed)
- No swelling
- No deformity
- Fall happened about 6 hours ago
- You can turn your wrist over
- There have been similar falls recently (you think it is careless tripping up)
- You need reassurance that arm not broken

Medical History

- Angina 8 years ago – Aspirin/Atenolol
- Osteo-arthritis of left hip 5 years ago – Co-codamol
- Symvastatin for cholesterol

Social Context

- Retired with large property to keep up to scratch
- Do all of cooking
- House has been adapted for wheelchair
- Go to swimming pool when wife has oxygen treatment every fortnight
- You normally drive – now worried about driving wife for treatment

Character

- Socially competent – handy around the house
- Take life as it comes
- Very chatty – like slipping out to talk to neighbours

Role-specific feedback

- [not appropriate for casualty]
- Dr expected to listen to present and past story
- Self-examination – history of previous falls
- Appropriate advice and painkillers

Example of information given to doctor

Call Information

Dennis Ruskin has just phoned (3.30pm) to say he fell and hurt his arm. He is worried that it is broken – feels he can't drive to the surgery and anyway can't leave his wife who has MS. Notes show angina (8 years ago) and hip problem. He is on Aspirin, Atenolol and Symvastatin. He attends irregularly himself, but frequently with wife.

Activity sequence

Confident that the telephone connection works and that the SPs have the schedule, the SP facilitator first checks experience among group members – those with experience may wish to determine a specific feedback focus. Experience of using SPs, the use of 'time out' etc. is also checked. They need to be aware that SPs will go silent on cue if there is a break in the consultation, in order that they can continue where they left off. The distinctive features of GP telephone consulting are then identified. There is a difference, for example, between a call made to an unknown nurse or doctor triage and one by a patient of the practice whose records will be on the screen (but not for this workshop). The absence of visual signals, the diagnostic uncertainty and the added complexity of decision making provide the reasoning behind the interlinked skills and abilities listed below: the one analytical, the other more personal. The call is made when the facilitator hands the Call Information from the receptionist to a group member.

Telephone consulting requires the development of the ability to:

- Spot emergencies
- Change expectations, i.e. give advice rather than visit
- Provide reassurance in the face of uncertainty
- Reassure anxious parents
- Avoid subsequent complaints (patients lack face to face messages!)

Specific skill requirements for telephone consultations

- Verbal cue sensitivity
- Identification of patient in-situ circumstances
- History taking that includes information normally obtained from observation or examination
- Risk assessment and prioritisation on verbal information alone, i.e. triaging
- Explicit safety netting

The fundamental issues above are discussed in an opportune manner as one telephone case follows another. The feedback dialogue after each case is enriched because observers are given the task of noting specific issues and interpersonal skills in use. At the conclusion of the session each group member is expected to develop their own interviewing guide with the help of the suggested headings:

Personal Telephone Interview Guideline* - Suggested headings

INTRODUCTION
Name exchange – kind of rapport – practice link

PATIENT'S CONTEXT
Location – support – who's listening in? - ICEE

SYMPTOM HISTORY
(Practitioner confidence to handle?)

OPTIONS & URGENCY

AGREED PLAN & SAFETY NET

DOUBLE CHECKING

*It is understood that a full range of interpersonal skills are required to fulfil this list.

The session can get very lively! One call involves a chatty woman, who some may classify as a time waster. How best to respond to her can arouse fierce debate, particularly when related to the time taken. Whether to visit a sick child or not can become very contentious, particularly after one very experienced GP told the group he always visits sick children.

Whether to send an elderly woman to hospital or not exposes one of the big uncertainties. She's waiting to go on holiday, but phones to check if her symptoms are serious. Indigestion is indicated, but at her age it might not be. The experienced GP, with safety in mind, advises that she be called in to check, but is it such a big risk? Particularly difficult is the case of a young woman refugee with limited English, whose symptoms tell of an infectious illness, but she refuses to take time off work because she depends upon her job in a burger bar to survive. What to do?

Options for all cases include: call the ambulance; go to hospital; home visit; immediate call-in (triage type decisions) or: advice and appointment; consultation with safety netting. The workshop emphasis is on the final option which of course involves full range proficiency.

Example of Patient Feedback Sheet

Patient .... Doctor ....

	Yes	No
I was able to tell the doctor about my problem(s)	Yes	No
I was not rushed	Yes	No
The doctor dealt with my concerns	Yes	No
My expectations were discussed	Yes	No
I could understand what the doctor said	Yes	No
I know what to do next	Yes	No

My thoughts and feelings about the consultation

Though based on a self-learner approach, facilitation of this workshop relies on an understanding that key features will be picked up and elaborated on opportunely, from one call to the next. After each call, feedback will follow the customary routine of caller feelings first, followed by observer reports on what's been heard and seen (it could be the caller's nervous posture). So much the better if opportunities for learning points emerge in this way. Otherwise the facilitator needs to challenge or expand on relevant issues. How do we know a particular patient is reassured, for instance?

Outcomes

Prior to the session's conclusion, time is set aside for silent reflection on what has been learnt. Thoughts are recorded on the Learning Capture Sheet as individual and general bullet points. These are then shared across the group. Hearing what colleagues have learnt adds another dimension to the workshop. The bullet points below have been selected from a collection of Learning Capture Sheets. It should be said that GPRs often make little distinction between individual and general points. Having omitted a repetition of common factors the list illuminates the wide range of personal learning from a standard workshop.

Individual Learning Points

Double check at end what patient understands

Expect the unexpected

I may go into too much detail on the telephone

Probably more useful if you do explore personal issues rather than wait until face-to-face

Get enough information, e,g, timescale of complaint

If you plan direct encounter – no need to spend time on the phone.

The threshold of doing a home visit seems lower than I'm used to?

Safety netting is most important when dealing with uncertainty

I learnt about interpersonal skills (list visible on charts)

'Listening' is vital – allowing time for patients to air their concerns – picking up verbal cues

Do not rush giving name and introductions

Use the word 'we' in forming management plans

On the phone patients cannot respond to my non-verbal communication so I need to make sure I'm vocalising empathy and remaining warm and approachable

Telephone consultations may feel longer than they really are

Useful analogies when explaining concepts to patients, e.g. motorways for nerves

General Learning Points

There are guidelines for non-face-to-face communication skills

Now I know a structured step by step plan (for telephone consultations)

Non-medical problems may be a prime concern

Learnt from listening to others react to different issues that we generally work the same

Useful to see others safety netting

Everyone can find telephone consulting difficult

At the end of the consultation the doctor and the patient need to be at ease with the decisions made

You rely very much on information given no matter how accurate it is

Get background/situation of patient

Usefulness of involving patients in own management plans

Summarise, Summarise, Summarise

Importance of taking a birth/neonatal history when assessing an ill child

Importance of 'house-keeping' after consultation

Confidentiality issues with possible listeners at the other end

Very difficult to break bad news over the phone – has patient support?

Megan Murray, an SP with many years' experience, presents workshops for the Simulated Patient Service and is Lead Simulator for the East Midlands GP Selection Centre. She played an integral part in the development of the Consultation Expertise Model, now a key feature of the Refreshing Consultation Skills workshop for GP practitioners.

Four

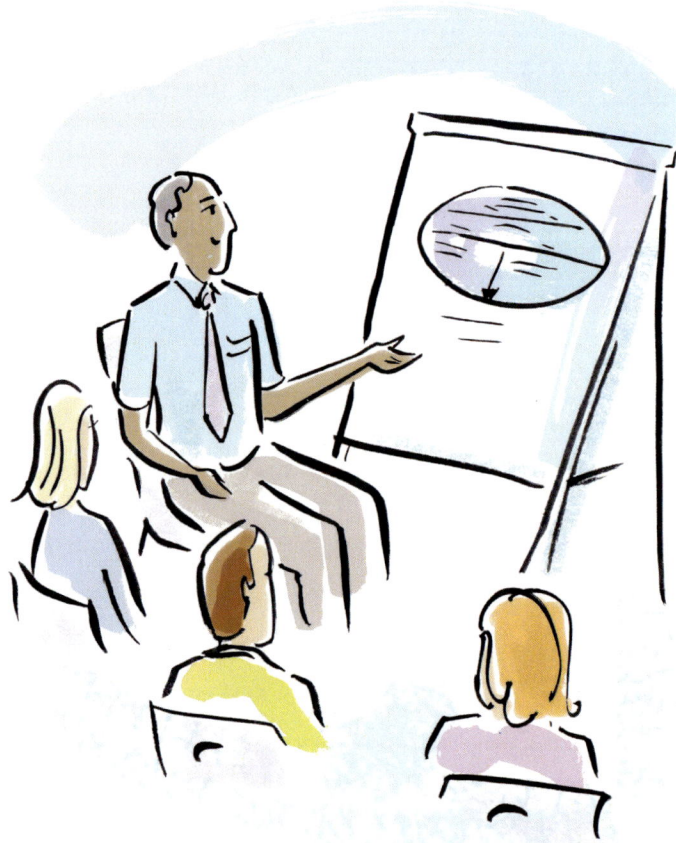

'Developing Therapeutic Rapport' Workshop

Reflections by Tim Norfolk

(The following is mostly transcribed directly from an interview, but includes some later clarifications by Tim)

What prompted the thinking behind the 'Developing Rapport' module?

For two years prior to developing that module I'd been involved with developing the new GP selection process, which had isolated six competencies to be assessed on the selection day (now incorporated into the National Selection Centre procedures). From that I began to develop the idea that there were three elements, three core skill areas.

Research Identifies GP Competencies (six assessed at selection centres)

- Empathy & Sensitivity

- Communication Skills

- Clinical Expertise

- Problem Solving

- Coping with Pressure

- Professional Integrity

One concerns eliciting information through empathy and communication skills; another analysing information using problem solving and clinical expertise; and a third, managing the situation and its specific pressures.

Skill Separation

Communication Skills
SURFACE (verbal & non-verbal)

Empathic Skills
DEEPER (cognitive/motivational)

The eliciting part is at the heart of the consultation, with its supporting literature around empathy. Researching empathy, I was struck by the fact that thinking had moved away from the idea of a felt experience – needing to feel what another person felt – to simply understanding what the other person felt, i.e. the cognitive side. This makes a lot more sense to me; if you understand, you don't have to feel, because the goal is to understand. But at the heart of understanding is first the motivation or desire to understand, and then the skills involved in asking questions and testing out ideas that emerge from what you've heard. This improves empathic accuracy (about the way someone is thinking or feeling). The only way you can ensure this is to have evidence from the other person that there is coherence between what you heard (or thought you heard) and what was actually said or intended.

The Empathic Journey

Empathic Motivation (desire to understand)
+
Empathic Attention (receptiveness)
+
Empathic Skill (making sense of clues)
⇨
Empathic Understanding (of patient perspective)
⇨
Therapeutic Rapport

So I proposed to Pat Lane (director of the South Yorkshire deanery) that I spend two years developing two of the essential three modules linked to key competencies for GP consultations: Developing Therapeutic Rapport and Problem Framing. (I later added the third, Shared Decision Making.)

Training Strategy (Day One)

Module One: Therapeutic Rapport

Morning

- Introduction to conceptual background
- 2 x consultation transcripts with role play
- 2 x video consultations
- Checklist of verbal and non-verbal signals

Afternoon

- 4 x simulated consultations in groups of 4/5 with specific observer tasks
- Feedback recorded on The Face

Day One was followed by a three-month period during which GP registrars would practise relevant skills and record outcomes in a work diary, then a follow-up half day when we met to explore progress made.

Was that so there would be a consistency between skills used to select doctors suitable as GP registrars and their subsequent training?

Absolutely; it was labelled as such – a two-year project aimed at developing the competencies required to be an effective GP. If you've selected people partly on the basis of empathy and communication skills then let's establish a well-grounded module that will develop those areas. If these are to be embedded as core skills then let's find a consistent way of developing them. That's how I became closely involved with the Leicester VTS and their simulators (having initially developed a link with the Leicester patch in 2000, when the new GP selection process was being piloted in the then Trent Deanery – with centres in Sheffield, Nottingham and Leicester).

It will be helpful if you would describe the thinking framework that underpins the model.

For me everything I do is a search for coherence. If things don't fit, they don't make sense – every process must be recognisable within some sort of pattern or framework. So within my initial 'eliciting, analysing & managing' jigsaw, the eliciting part involved a very specific interaction between empathy and communication skills. I know you (Peter) talk often about using empathy as one element in eliciting the patient's story, but to me this is too often defined simply by the use of easily identifiable communication skills rather than deeper empathic skills. These facilitating verbal and non-verbal behaviours do form a distinct part of my model of developing rapport but they are in an important sense secondary to the underlying empathic journey. Anything to do with smiling, nodding, facilitative phrasing, echoing, etc – these are simply techniques. They don't have any intrinsic meaning in themselves. Their effectiveness is ultimately dependent on the quality of empathic understanding they serve as 'tools' to generate.

In the now widely accepted definition of empathy, the starting point is one's motivation – the desire to understand. There are a lot of people, including some GPs, who aren't really that interested in what the other person is thinking or feeling about their situation or problem. And if you're not really interested, the other person's brain 'clocks' that message; you then don't fully attend to the situation, and shouldn't be surprised if you miss potentially important signals or cues. So empathy is initially about the motivation. There are two inherent or innate trait elements – warmth and/or curiosity – which can drive that process. If you are low on both counts you're in trouble, though you can

in the short-term draw on professional integrity by telling yourself it's *important* to care and therefore to listen. The motivational factor is then backed up by the skill – the empathic skill of being able to accurately identify and analyse a patient's thoughts and feelings about their problem.

That's an important qualification for SPs who've been party to the acquisition of interpersonal skills, starting with open and closed questions in the medical school on to the more sophisticated skills necessary to include aspects of patients' 'lifeworld' in a more holistic consultation. You're saying we've missed a key skill?

Yes, the core skills associated with the effective demonstration of empathy are diagnostic, merely supported by the communication skills. Assessing a patient's thoughts and feelings involves the same search for specific and identifiable information as the clinician looking at someone's knee or listening to them talking about a skin complaint. The patient says, 'It's been a bit of a struggle because of this and that', you hear the sigh or see the tightening of the facial expression – and a similar diagnostic journey is underway. Identifying and putting those pieces together is in essence an analytical process much in the same way as any biomedical exploration. Empathic skills are the internal heartland of rapport building, and communication skills merely 'oil' that interactive search for understanding and personal meaning. Thus the way you ask a question, the way you respond, the way you smile, the way you look – these facilitate or enable a patient's primary thoughts and feelings to be articulated; they encourage openness, but they are not of themselves to do with empathy – and for me, it's a crucial distinction. You are working on two skill-sets.

The problem is you find a lot of people who use communication skills fluently but fail to analyse effectively; they miss the point. They use them formulaically. And when they 'miss a cue', they make a classic diagnostic error. For me training is too often misdirected in terms of the skill area that is being addressed and why. When I set up the module, I was very clear that the first part (day one; the full day) involved a deep grounding in what it means to be empathic. That requires some initially overt 'teaching'.

You have to tell them what the context is?

Absolutely. For me, that's the cognitive element – to ensure they fully understand the process involved in searching for that central goal of therapeutic rapport. Until somebody properly understands what is involved, what is required, they can't direct their attention and efforts in a way that is rational and meaningful enough for them to build a structure upon; of course, that's presuming they have access to the wider cognitive awareness guiding the skills – i.e. the metacognition!

What you've been explaining so lucidly is a precursor to the model as I now think of it. But how do you achieve that 'wider cognitive awareness' in practice?

The video recording is crucial – it enables me to explain the language of empathy. It is a recording of two SPs, Martin and Dina, consulting as doctor and patient. It should be the masterstroke of every training session. They do two versions. In the first, Dina plays the doctor in a rather cold, formulaic consultation. In the second she switches gears and starts eliciting and responding to cues and clues (there is a distinction!). We then compare the two versions and finally I ask the group where they think Dina is relative to their own current training level. They typically say maybe 3rd year, maybe even beyond. I pause and say, 'That's very interesting… because what you've seen is actually a lawyer who only saw the case half an hour before'. They go completely silent. It

blows the myth out of the water – the myth that there is something mystical about a medic communicating with a patient. That's a classic late morning 'shake' to the system. So they go to lunch with a somewhat difficult truth to absorb and reflect on.

What were the simulators asked to do?

Both modules were presented with close attention to detail, be it for doctors, trainers, facilitators or simulators, i.e. with paper instructions for every stage. The SP scenarios for this module were adapted from ICE workshops run by the Leicester Simulated Patient Unit, so the SPs only had to absorb detail new to them. The small group workshops with 4 to 5 GPRs were often led by the trainers/facilitators but also sometimes (especially latterly) self-facilitated by the SPs – an interesting opportunity for the patient experience to be fully central to the training session. They were expected to follow this tightly-timed procedure and incorporate an extended understanding of empathic and communication skills:

SP tasks for each 15-minute session (consultation & feedback)

- Identify doctor/consultor
- Allocate observer roles
- SIMULATE PATIENT CASE for 4 minutes
- Allow 2 minutes of reflection time
- Guide observers (and consultor) through recording of perceptions of patient's thoughts/feelings & verbal/non-verbal behaviours on The Face diagram
- Disclose patient's actual thoughts and feelings
- Discuss differences

Observers' non-verbal patient & doctor behaviour prompts

- Facial expression (smiling, frowning, expressionless etc)
- Nodding
- Eye contact
- Vocal patterns (volume, tone, pitch, pace)
- Hand gestures
- Posture (leaning forward/backward, legs open/crossed)
- Movement (arms, legs, feet, body…)
- Any MIRRORING of patient non-verbal behaviour (especially vocal patterns)
- Any adjustment of non-verbal behaviour (esp. vocal)

Case – Kenneth Scoresby age 66

Mr Scoresby attends at the doctor's request for a review of change of bowel function. He is known to have diverticular disease. He has been depressed in the past and is feeling stressed at the moment. He has taken on too much at church just when his wife has major surgery. His personal strategy has led to improvements. He does not consider himself depressed, but will concede likely symptoms. He does not wish to take medication.

Part of the underlying theme of the module is that you don't need a 10 minute simulated exercise to prove the point around empathy; you only need the 'golden minute', so doctors have 4 minutes to establish a connection.

The Patient Face

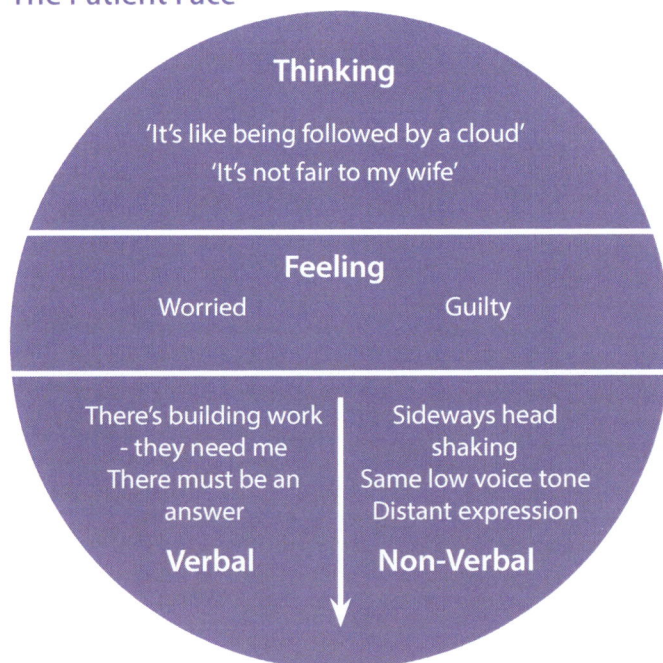

Thinking

'It's like being followed by a cloud'
'It's not fair to my wife'

Feeling

Worried   Guilty

There's building work - they need me
There must be an answer

Sideways head shaking
Same low voice tone
Distant expression

Verbal   **Non-Verbal**

The feedback concludes with a comparison of the evidence behind the patient 'face' and the declared patient's thoughts and feelings.

Kenneth Scoresby

Thoughts

- The doctor will know what is wrong with me
- I ought to be able to sort myself out – maybe I/we need a break
- Will the burden get worse?
- I'm not being fair to Margaret
- I'm letting the church down

Feelings

- Feeling down
- Confusion
- Worry
- Guilt

So, you were extending the well-entrenched ICE formula?

Yes, but we had an interesting dialogue while I was trying to persuade you guys to deconstruct it. That was because the concerns discussed are typically ideas rather than feelings (and that's the flaw in the ICE terminology!). The challenge for the trainee – and this has now been modelled in CSA – is to elicit the core thoughts and feelings of each patient. Try to get as clear an understanding as you can of where someone is coming from; chase the heat; find out what is at the heart of that person's story. So, the SPs were asked, as they are now in CSA, to be responsive to the way in which the doctor was dealing with them. If someone appears to be 'facilitating' you, enabling you, release more. There's 4 minutes and you then have a period of reflection in which the patient, observers and trainee make notes. Crucially, during the session the observers were recording verbal and non-verbal behaviour. We were modelling the 'ORCE' process (the standard process for behaviour assessment in occupational psychology).

1. Observe, record, classify, evaluate (ORCE). We had that period of silent reflection afterwards when everybody wrote down what they'd gleaned from those 4 minutes in terms of evidence. This was followed by a sequence of feedback from patient, doctor, and then from observers – the ALOBA feedback process.

2. The big moment is the simulator's feedback. Everything hinges on that – the 'patients' must go last. I wanted anybody who might be complacent to test their assumptions both as doctors and observers. So often they assume that they've nailed it. Then the patient comes in and says, 'Early on I hesitated and said I wasn't quite sure, but that wasn't picked up'.

3. For me everything comes down to the unambiguous verbal and non-verbal

evidence. I wanted to deconstruct the myth with the empathy work and with the practice module – the myth that there was something that couldn't be defined. For me, everything can be defined. What was happening was entirely accessible or recognisable: there was evidence, and you either get the evidence or you don't.

4. The feedback was constructed so the GPRs all had to table their perceptions first (whether consultor or observer), without any hints from the patient. By holding the 'patient' until last, the GPRs couldn't hide potential weaknesses or flawed perceptions – otherwise the opportunity to learn and adapt current practice is lost. I didn't want any ambiguity; it was crucial to me that the SPs, when trained up, knew and owned the specific thoughts and feelings associated with their particular presentation or problem, and didn't lose track of that.

Presumably, SPs could express themselves differently according to the nature of the consultation?

Yes. Ideally they would later say something like, 'Because of the journey I was taken on, my thoughts moved' - or not! For example, 'I wasn't able to articulate that thought', or, 'I became anxious and a new thought came', or, 'I became more reassured and that thought was eased', (i.e. specific to their presenting thoughts and feelings). Thereafter, the degree to which the patient feels understood will determine the degree to which they'll get involved in the negotiation that follows.

It seems to me that while you've been constructing a post-ICE model by defining and incorporating the cognitive elements of empathy, you have also paved the way for a more integrative understanding of clinical expertise – one that subsumes interpersonal skills. Would you agree?

Indirectly, I guess that's possible – in terms of widening discussion of a doctor's disciplined 'diagnostic' skills to include the search for psychosocial meaning, seeing the latter as demanding a parallel rigour and recognisable process rather than relying on (or presuming that) empathic understanding or therapeutic rapport can only happen through some sort of mystical or 'natural' flow between doctor or patient. In the hands of a highly gifted consultor there can indeed seem to be an effortless, spontaneous dynamic going on, where the eliciting by doctor and 'revealing' by patient happen seamlessly, and an almost immediate and lasting rapport is established. This does happen. But it's not remotely the norm, and for most doctors empathic understanding is a challenging goal – demanding deliberate, self-conscious learning, repeated practice and honest reflection.

Tim Norfolk is an independent occupational psychologist.

Extracted from: Developing therapeutic rapport: a training validation study

By Tim Norfolk, Kamaljit Birdi, Fiona Patterson
Quality in Primary Care 2009; 17:99-106

Research Background

The specific aim of the study was to evaluate the potential of a short-term training programme using this model to improve rapport-related behaviour in general practitioner (GP) trainees.

Results

The training group demonstrated significant increases in rapport-related knowledge and all three affective dimensions (attitudes, confidence and motivation); there was a similar finding in terms of 'positive engagement' and all expert-rated aspects of rapport-related behaviours. The control group showed no comparable improvement in any area, and recorded a significant drop in demonstration of positive engagement behaviours.

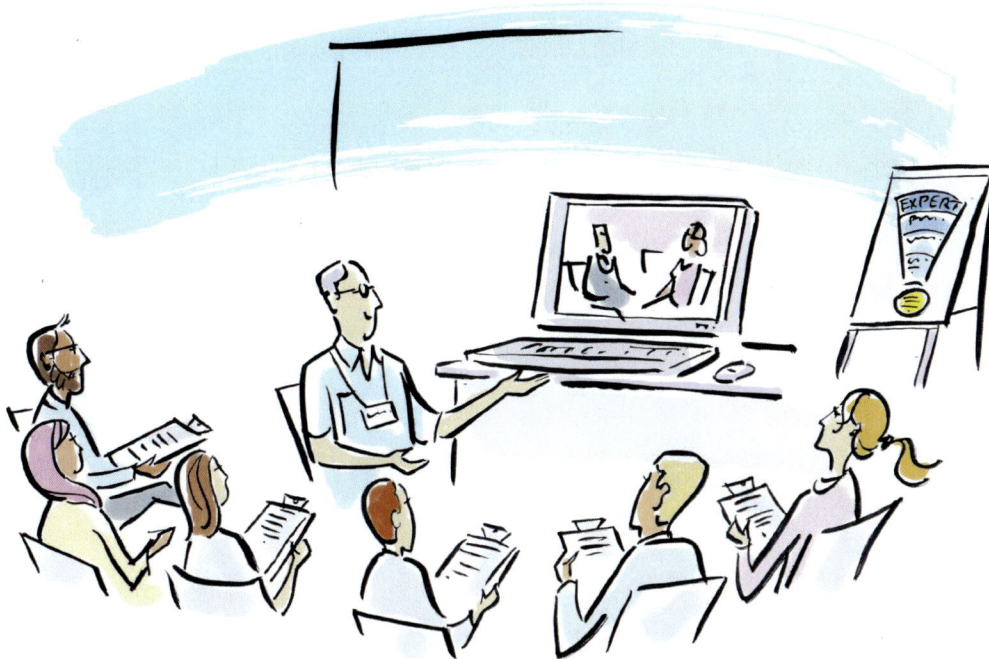

Refreshing Consultation Skills Workshop for GP Practioners

A Report

Origins

The Refreshing Consultation Skills workshop uses the Consultation Expertise Model (CEM) as a guide to frame learning activity. CEM was developed over many years by practicing GPs to identify what higher-order consulting expertise looks like in day-to-day practice. It considers what happens between doctor and patient according to the eight *domain* headings on the next page. Radiating from the *consulting skills* centre there are a series of *indicative statements* for each *domain* at three expertise levels – *competent / proficient / expert*. Using CEM, GPs can judge the level of expertise in any one consultation by making a diagrammatic *fingerprint*. That's if they have the tenacity to record the consultation and identify the level of behaviour in some or all of the domains. When we've tried to explain the model, designed, as it is, for practitioner self-use, colleagues have told us they are bemused by the amount of detail.

To address this, we contemplated devising a teaching programme based on three 'expert' common factors, identified in experienced GP consultations. The doctors in these consultations appeared to 'start anywhere', 'go there', and achieve 'concordant' outcomes – three reductive labels for complex and idiosyncratic behaviour – a simplification of complex behaviour[1].

Fortunately, these common factors can be explored practically with simulated patients, and thereafter taken to signify essential attributes of a complete consultation as well as lead-ins to CEM. From this starting point, together with a generous grant from the East Midlands Healthcare Workforce Deanery, we developed the pilot workshop.

---

[1] I am only interested in simplicity on the other side of complexity. This axiom suggests that there are three stages of knowledge. The first level is simplicity born of ignorance, as when someone says, 'Oh that's simple', but doesn't know what they are talking about. The second level is complexity born of understanding – when you realize a subject is far more complex than it first appears on the surface. The third is simplicity born of the profound. **Fred Lee**, *If Disney Ran Your Hospital: 9½ Things You Would Do Differently.*

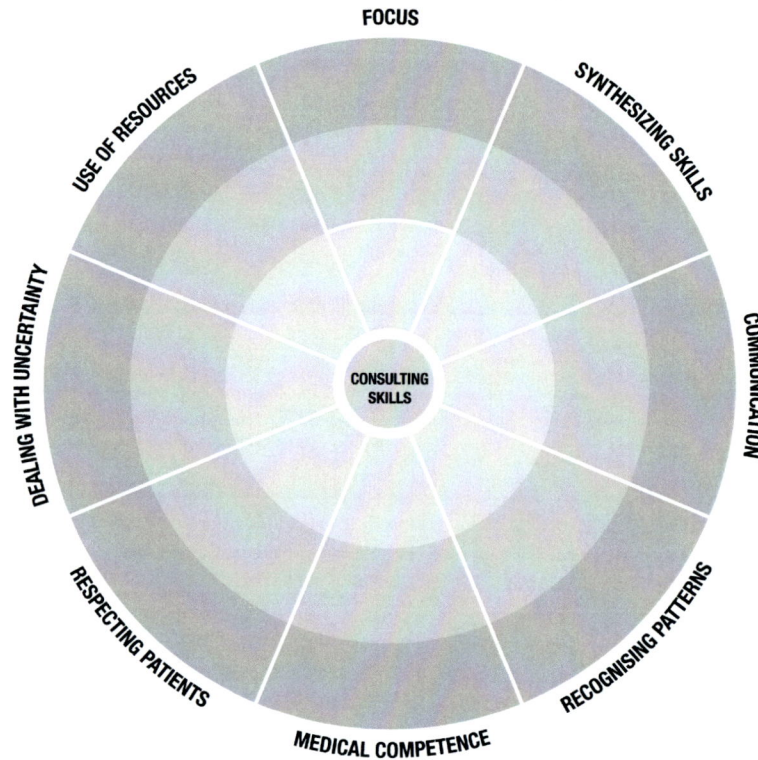

Bevis Heap
Learning Purpose

FOCUS

SYNTHESIZING SKILLS

USE OF RESOURCES

DEALING WITH UNCERTAINTY

Rhiannon Prytherch
Simulation

CONSULTING
SKILLS

COMMUNICATION

Phil Rayner
Facilitation

RESPECTING PATIENTS

RECOGNISING PATTERNS

MEDICAL COMPETENCE

Megan Murray
Presentation and development

Pilot workshop

With the CEM as the learning framework for three GP facilitated groups of four practitioners each, the pilot had all the features of our customary SP workshops, but because we were exploring how to refine the workshop for future use, on this first occasion we had two GP facilitators for each small group and nine different SP cases – all developed from real patient consultations according to the Leicester method. This was the first time we, as a team, had organised this kind of workshop for GP practitioners, some of whom came with a lifetime of unobserved consulting, some of whom were still in their first three years of practice. Surprisingly it worked, but cost-wise it was unrepeatable.

The evaluation by an experienced educational inspector endorsed the effectiveness of basing the workshop around the three attributes. Surprisingly, *flexibility* was exposed as an additional attribute for expertise development, which was perhaps an inevitable consequence of 'starting anywhere'. Lots of other issues surfaced: the difficulty of facilitating experienced GPs with such a wide range of experience, simpler use of domain paperwork, and the related question of how best to link CEM purpose and statements to what is going on with the patient. In this respect, simulators were found to provide active value throughout. The pilot provided an encouraging start as well as highlighting areas for adjustment. In terms of learning purpose, the evaluator found:

'All [participants] testified to the value of the professional development opportunity, in particular the appreciation and application through simulations of the Consultation Expertise Model (CEM) as a means of learning how to improve a core practice – consulting with patients – that is the centrepiece of their work.'

From evaluation conducted by Brian Merton

An ever recurring issue concerns our ability to sustain sufficient trust with disparate groups of GP practitioners in order to gain benefit from group-work with SPs.

Presentation and development of workshop structure

A distinctive feature of the workshop is the conjunction of SP presentation with GP group facilitation – our SP presenter was involved in the research stage of CEM and so comes with an intimate knowledge of the model! Through delivering the workshops, she has been instrumental in their development. This has involved the design and production of faculty and group training material, liaising with facilitators and SPs and with those who commission the workshops; presently that's the GP appraisal team operating within Leicestershire and Leicester city. For each workshop she presents the introduction and keeps an overview on what's happening from session to session, i.e. keeping track of time and delegates' experience. At the end she collects the feedback and collates it for review with the team.

Workshop process

At first the workshops took a whole day. Currently they start at 1pm and finish at 7.30pm. As we are mindful that people come from a busy morning surgery, we give them time to settle in and have lunch. Delegates range from those recently qualified to those coming up to retirement. A number have been appraisers. Amongst the GPs are some who may have been advised to come on the back of an appraisal. In one or two instances complaints from patients have prompted attendance. We've worked very hard to establish a safe, supportive and confidential environment. To that end we headline the fact that using CEM has nothing at all to do with assessment; *we're here to celebrate people's consulting.*

We explain how delegates may benefit from working in a group with SPs. It's often new for some delegates. Stopping, restarting, reviewing, rewinding and then receiving feedback from colleagues and facilitators – a key part of the workshop – can be a challenging leap from normal weekday practice. After scrutinising the introductory DVD with its emphasis on identifying *expertise*, each of the two groups have three SP sessions focused on the three attributes, during which time volunteers consult with a range of patient cases. For the first session on 'starting anywhere' the consultation is stopped after 2 minutes in order to focus on the initial interaction. Ideally, the consultor and other volunteers will then try different approaches that challenge the 'what can I do for you today' kind of habit. The emphasis throughout is on the opportunity to refresh consulting by trying different approaches.

Workshop content - introducing CEM

At the beginning we play a recording of a very experienced GP consulting with a diabetic patient. Delegates are asked to identify what they see as examples of *advanced* consulting, exclusively from what the doctor is saying and doing. This provides evidence to support their ideas of what advanced consulting looks like and, later, how these ideas are encapsulated within the model.

We stress that the model is simply a different way to look at what can happen every day, in a manner consistent with previous practice. From that shared understanding we can highlight the reasoning behind the three attributes we explore in each session. The three attributes provide a lead-in to the model, and, as we are prone to reinforce, serve as prompts for reflection in day-to-day practice.

This can be illustrated with evidence from the recorded consultation. For example, someone might say the GP picked up a cue and acknowledged it by using the same language as the patient – indeed mirrored the patient and used that cue throughout the consultation. The GP has entered the patient's 'lifeworld'. In the recorded example, we find that the patient's wife is suffering from depression – by picking this up it becomes possible to explore how the wife's condition is impacting on the patient's health.

We can then map back from an attribute – here it's the doctor 'going there' i.e. exploring the patient's 'lifeworld' – to indicative statements in one of the CEM domains, and thereby to levels of expertise, as can be seen in the below example.

Going There

Example of Link with Indicative Statements

CEM DOMAIN – Synthesising Skills

Competent: Tends to be doctor-centred

Proficient: Responds appropriately to emotion in the consultation

Expert: Uses emotional affect of the patient as a diagnostic tool

The recorded consultation, though relaxed and conversational, as with most expert consultations, clearly shows how 'starting anywhere', maps into 'going there' and then onto 'concordance'. There's quite a lot of evidence on the recording to show how the patient and the GP move towards an agreed management plan. So, while that helps us demonstrate the three attributes rationale, it's also possible to underline how observed behaviour can be traced back to the eight domains.

'Starting anywhere'

We recognise how difficult it can be to adapt, or to adapt an habitual consulting style. But it's at such moments, outside the comfort zone, when light bulbs can go on. 'Starting anywhere' provides an interesting example. During feedback, one delegate wrote, 'If you don't say anything, it can reveal all sorts of things about the patient'; a dramatic move away from the formulaic, 'What can I do for you today'.

While focused on the start of the consultation, 'starting anywhere' is about settling into the group work as well; it gives the facilitator a chance to establish feedback guidelines. One of the desired outcomes is that delegates will become familiar with the CEM and will start to use it from the very beginning. To that end, we pick out domains. Looking at the communication domain by itself, this translates as 'the doctor will encourage the patient to respond' at the expert level, and 'accepts things at face value' at the competent level.

At the end of the day delegates will have experienced four different consultations, become familiar with the three attributes and the way they link to domain statements, been observed by their peers, and received feedback. Their performance will be shown as part of or a whole fingerprint – a snapshot of where they sit on the competent, proficient and expert levels.

Starting Anywhere

Example of Link with Indicative Statements

CEM DOMAIN – Respecting Patients

Competent: Acknowledges patient

Proficient: Copes with the patient and their problems

Expert: Works with the individuality of the patient

Previously we've ended with each small group reflecting on the day's learning and then comparing each group's learning points in whole group discussion. We've now introduced an additional SP consultation. After one delegate volunteers to do an uninterrupted consultation we distribute the domain sheets amongst the observers. By identifying the indicative statements in each domain, we end up with a complete fingerprint for that consultation.

End of workshop evaluation

At the end we ask whether delegates have had a meaningful introduction to CEM and whether they are familiar enough to use it. By and large there is agreement that we have met the outcomes; that's with a degree of ambivalence about using CEM subsequently for appraisal or revalidation. It's seen as something of a luxury given current demands on GPs' time. Happily, there is usually an interpersonal skill bi-product from observing colleagues and working with SPs, e.g. 'I saw how valuable it is to summarise, not just at the end but at key points during the consultation'.

Group facilitation

From the outset it was clear that facilitating disparate groups of GP practitioners demands previous experience. Experience whereby the skill of *going over the ground rules* and *dealing with quiet and dominant members* is taken for granted. Most important in groups where there is continuity such as with GP registrars and trainers is *allowing the group to direct where their learning goes*. Phil Rayner recollects, *I remember one group in which it had become apparent there were no activists, but their task was to devise a presentation. I parked myself in the group circle and said nothing. It worked, someone took the initiative. With experience, I now feel more confident that I don't need to prepare everything in detail; better to let the group generate its own*

momentum – sometimes that's more easily said than done!

The *Refreshing* groups are one-offs with delegates of different age and experience. Getting experienced GPs to think about what they are doing and why they are doing it that way, while recognising that others might do things a bit differently, becomes a priority. That alternative strategies might work better is a workshop sub-text. Then there is the question of what you do with someone who is struggling. Some may go away with two or three new skills, while others who are not on the same wavelength won't do anything different. With CEM you are dipping your toes in a pond with lots of depths. 'Starting anywhere', 'going there' and 'concordance' are simple starting points and that's what some will go away with. Go beyond that – by exploring the patient's 'lifeworld'; and looking at how your interpersonal and clinical skills match up with CEM domains – and you are in another world.

For some, even going into the patient's lifeworld is new. Even for those who are well practiced at switching from doctor-centred to patient-centred mode, the domains can appear complicated. It's vital that everyone becomes involved. The small group works fine when the SPs can switch from one role to another. They are very believable, authentic and challenging. Without the opportunity to practise delegate's skills this course would not be effective. It tests facilitator skills as well! For example, feedback is crucial to the learning but despite forthright advice to follow feedback rules, some will always ask the SP for value based feedback, of the 'how did I do?' variety. That's very frustrating because access to the indicative statements depends entirely on the behaviours that are seen, heard and can be recalled. Those types of question present SPs with a feedback dilemma if they are to respond in role.

Concordance

Example of link with Indicative Statements

Domain – Dealing with Uncertainty

Competent: Recognises where there is uncertainty and risk but doesn't share this with the patient

Proficient: Introduces uncertainty (with attendant risk) about diagnosis and management

Expert: Where necessary uses uncertainty as a starting point for negotiating with the patient

'Concordance' requires a patient-centred approach

Most difficult is the realisation that someone is not very competent; how is that to be fed back? The only hope is that the light bulb will go on when it's realised they are not consulting the way others are. Maybe the bulb will switch on when they go away and think about it.

Doctors always tell you what they would like to do differently but they are not good at seeking out things they do well. CEM works on evidence – what did he say – what did you see? Having your peer group observe you and point out when higher levels are achieved can be very affirming. Furthermore, realising that you are hitting expert level in certain domains is uniquely reinforcing. How often does this happen in day-to-day practice?

With GPRs and fellow trainers there is an assumption that activity is there to help them. With GP practitioners the mandate is fuzzier. Some come to compare their already proficient consulting. On the other hand, one doctor who was getting patient complaints wanted to understand what he was doing wrong. It soon became clear why he was upsetting his patients

so he was able to do something about it. Some only come to tick the CPD box. That said, feedback on the day is generally very positive; there aren't many opportunities for established GPs to reflect on their consulting these days.

How GPs might benefit in future from CEM we do not know. Maybe the initial recording with its modelling of how a high quality consultation can be achieved well within ten minutes will be recalled. What is manifestly clear is the value of observing colleagues consulting with the SP cases and unpicking what happened in the context of a high expectation model.

Refreshing consultation skills with patient simulations

Nine cases and nine SPs were used for the pilot workshop. This has been reduced to five cases and two SPs – each SP now presents two or three cases – a task which requires very experienced simulators to retain patient authenticity. The reduction in personnel has been made possible by splitting the number of delegates into two groups of six and incorporating the 'starting anywhere' session into the introduction.

SP case example presented by Rhiannon Prytherch

L.S. is a Leicester method role, recorded specifically for Refreshing the Consultation. She has proved to be a suitable case to explore the three attributes. Her previous medical history is provided for the consultor. In brief, she attends because it seems she's getting depressed again but doesn't want medication. Having recovered from her previous low mood she now has a job in a care home where she felt obliged to complain to her supervisor about the way inmates were being treated. Regarded as a whistle blower she has subsequently been cold shouldered by fellow workers. A single mum, she is also worried about her teenage son's dislocated lifestyle. As she is fully aware of her condition she doesn't come for an expert diagnosis. It's a perfect role when it comes to the concordance, if that side of her character is embraced.

As Rhiannon says, *the consultation is very much about picking up nonverbal cues. There are lots of silences which I use to emphasise the fact that I don't look happy.* Nor does she respond quickly. L.S clearly does not want to go down the depression route. As some doctors try to go down that route, L.S. reacts according to what they do. This is regarded as *behaviour that breeds behaviour.* Reflecting on her experience with this workshop – a very intense six hours – Rhiannon identifies three issues:

Personalisation sensitivity

One is a hyper awareness of how she personalises a role. If she is not careful she can change the case priority for the doctor. For example, a depressed patient may not be suicidal but minor hints could take it down that route. Ever since the second E was added to ICE she has been sensitive to the fact that doctors may offer more support to someone like L.S. who's having a miserable time on her own, than they may offer to someone with family up the road with a wonderful husband. Such details can easily change a consultation, particularly if the purpose is to explore 'going there'. With the Refreshing workshop *it's not about us, it's about doctors and their learning. It doesn't matter if the scenario is not 100% authentic as long as delegates get the key learning points in a way they can respond to and engage with.* In this she retains the validity of the 'patient voice' alongside an awareness of the three attributes link to CEM for feedback, which in turn helps her to avoid personalisation distractions.

Sensing patient-centred consulting

CEM is very much a patient-centred model. Rhiannon has become very sensitive that starting anywhere involves having the bravery to let go and follow her story. When she brings up her initial, 'This is why I've come', doctors <u>can</u> start anywhere. She says, *patient-centredness goes all the way through. For instance, I love the fact that it's called concordance – in lots of other clinical education situations I hear it called management. To me that implies there's a problem that needs managing from the outside, which implies the removal of some responsibility from the patient.* She knows intuitively when the delegate's agenda is uppermost and when they want to finish the case quickly to make it easier for them.

Responding and feedback

SPs are a means to understanding the model and its implications for consulting practice. But it's the facilitators who unlock the way SPs respond; mainly through the way they guide requests for feedback. Rhiannon recalls one doctor, who was struggling with 'starting anywhere'. He hadn't noticed that she was sitting there with arms closed, avoiding eye contact. He still asked, 'How did I do? To which her answer was a shrug. He couldn't phrase a question that would elicit the reason for her response; if asked, she would have told him, *I felt you were ignoring me!* SPs rely on facilitators to unplug that kind of difficulty. *Only questions based on specific observations of what happened and what was felt by me, the patient, can be related back to the model.*

Rhiannon reflects: *it's best when facilitators bring us in as the third party after they have unpacked what the candidate did and how that ties in with the model. How did it feel for you – how reassured did you feel about the agreed treatment? Those questions have a dual purpose. They have to refer to the model, but also through the simulator where possible. The simulator strengthens it. Mind you, facilitators do get presented with problematic colleagues. We had an 'eye-closer' once. What do they do about that?*

Sometimes the openness to learning is not there. I don't mean that in a bad way as if they are closed off to learning. They are simply out of practice and engaging with a whole new model is not easy. This is where peer-observers, facilitators and SPs can really help.

Dr Bevis Heap and Dr Phil Rayner are practicing GPs who train GP registrars in their practices and also work as Programme Directors for the wider vocational training scheme. Rhiannon Prytherch is a widely experienced SP as is Megan Murray who also presents workshops.

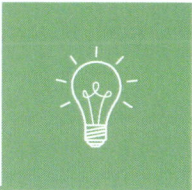

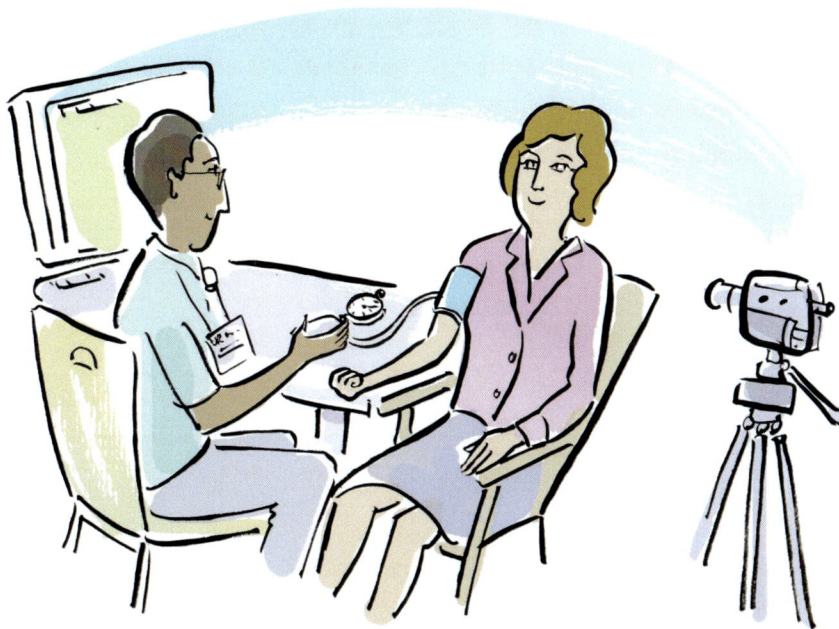

Using Simulated Patients for Research

Conversations with Adrian French and Carolyn Oldershaw

Background

This is the story of how an enquiry by a group of eight local doctors and two non-clinical educators developed a means to identify the nature of high level expertise in general practice consulting. At each stage, the enquiry was carried forward by the use of simulated patients.

An awareness of the enquiry outcome, the Consultation Expertise Model (CEM), will be helpful in illustrating the part played by SPs. The enquiry developed over several years and was initially more like a hobby than a research project. That said, the question driving the enquiry – **what distinguishes the consulting behaviour of more experienced GPs** – was considered to be on a previously unexplored frontier.

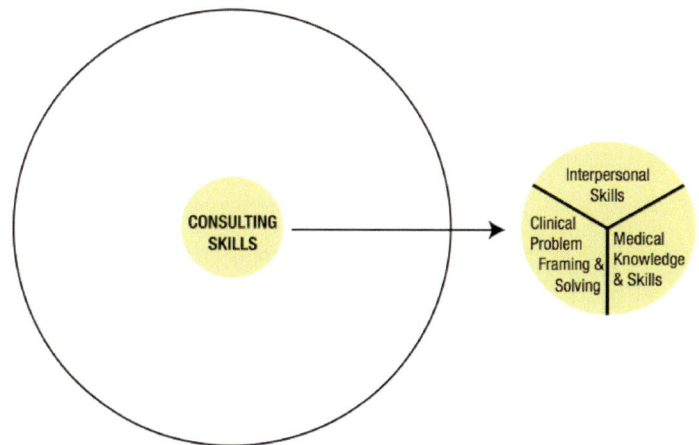

Core Consulting Skills

- Medical knowledge and skills
- Clinical problem framing and solving
- Interpersonal skills

Figure 1 - Three Core Consulting Skills

The Consultation Expertise Model (CEM) is presented as a circular diagram with Consulting Skills at its core (Figure 1)

Consulting Domains

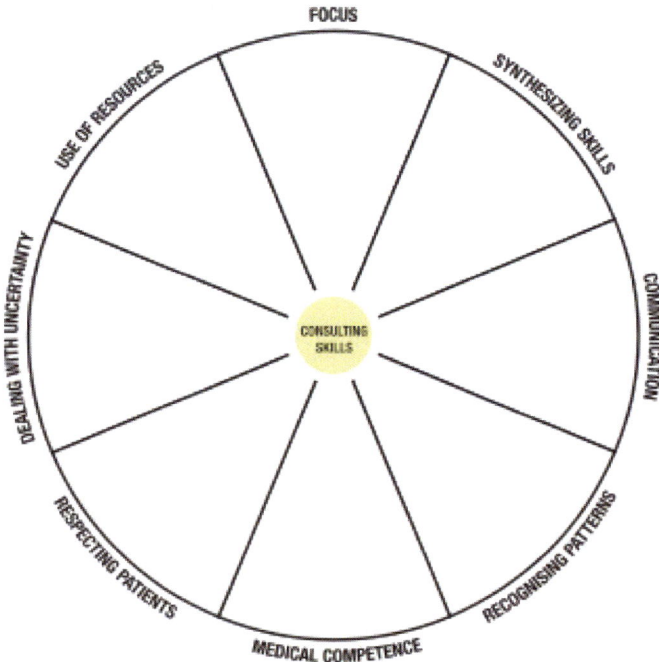

- Communication
- Recognising Patterns
- Medical Competence
- Respecting Patients
- Dealing with Uncertainty
- Use of Resources
- Focus
- Synthesising Skills

Figure 2 – Eight Consulting Domains

The circle is further split into eight segments referred to as Domains, each representing an aspect of general practitioner behaviour (Figure 2). It must be emphasised that this is for analytical purposes only. Doctors do not think like this while consulting!

Expertise Levels

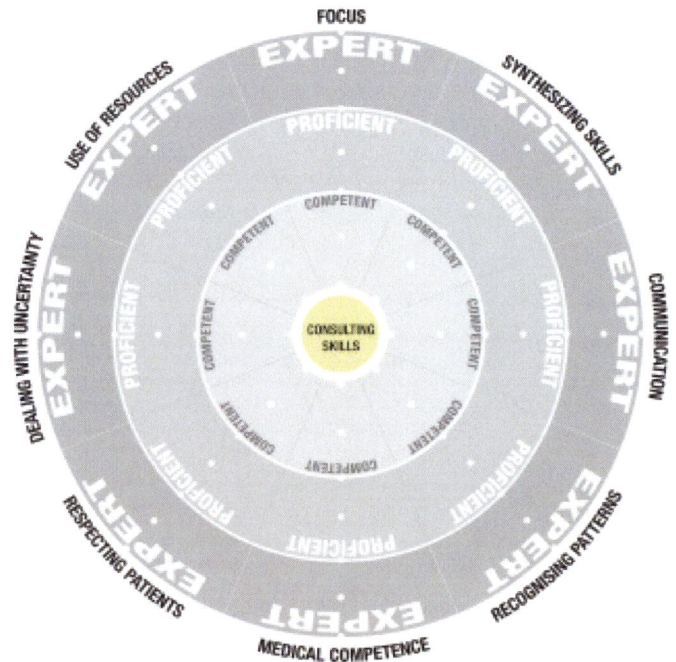

- Competent
- Proficient
- Expert

Figure 3 – Three Expertise Levels

In order to recognise different consulting Expertise Levels, three quality identifiers radiate from the core (Figure 3)

At this point in its development CEM is a model of little use.

Indicative Statements

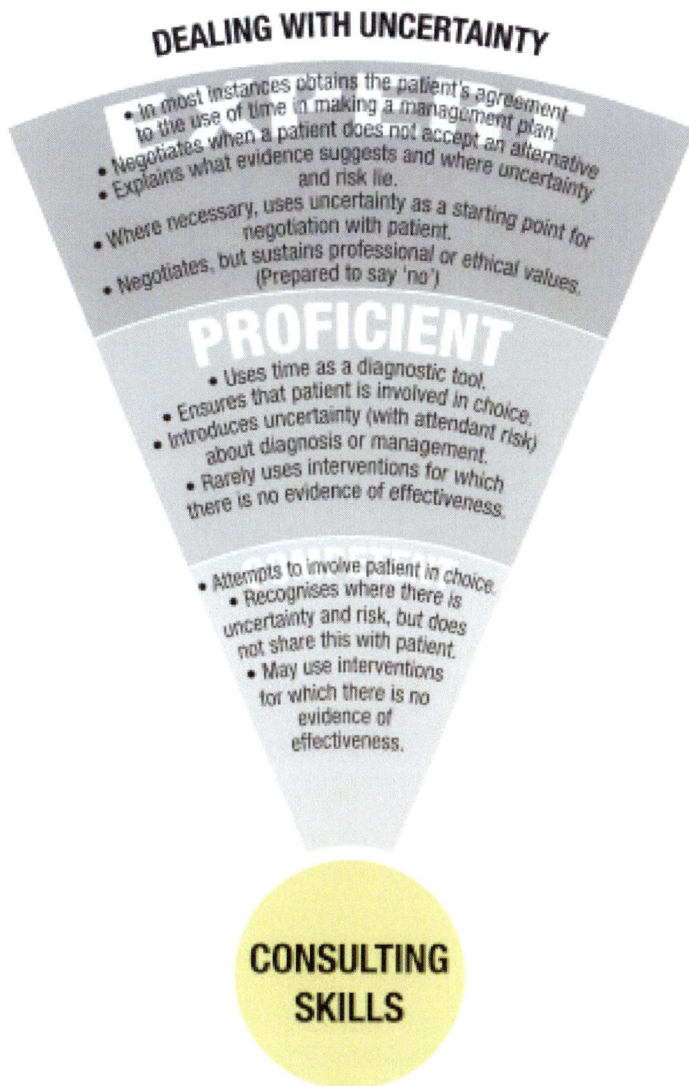

DEALING WITH UNCERTAINTY

EXPERT
- In most instances obtains the patient's agreement to the use of time in making a management plan.
- Negotiates when a patient does not accept an alternative
- Explains what evidence suggests and where uncertainty and risk lie.
- Where necessary, uses uncertainty as a starting point for negotiation with patient.
- Negotiates, but sustains professional or ethical values. (Prepared to say 'no')

PROFICIENT
- Uses time as a diagnostic tool.
- Ensures that patient is involved in choice.
- Introduces uncertainty (with attendant risk) about diagnosis or management.
- Rarely uses interventions for which there is no evidence of effectiveness.

- Attempts to involve patient in choice.
- Recognises where there is uncertainty and risk, but does not share this with patient.
- May use interventions for which there is no evidence of effectiveness.

CONSULTING SKILLS

One Indicative Statement at expert level for Dealing with Uncertainty provides an example:

- Explains what evidence suggests and where uncertainty and risk lie.

Figure 4 - Indicative Statements for Each Domain

It is the addition of Indicative Statements – example Figure 4 above – that provides the detail with which to identify expertise levels in each domain in order to record them as an expertise case Fingerprint – Figure 5 next.

Case Fingerprints

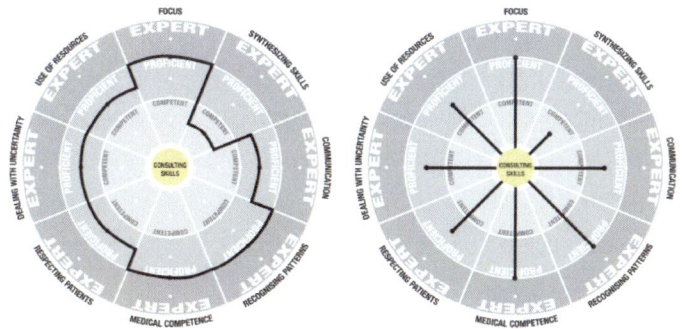

- At a glance this fingerprint indicates overall proficiency with three domains at the proficient/expert boundary. Curiously, Synthesising Skills registers as competent. This may be because of case aspects but for whatever reason, it can prompt discussion.

Figure 5 shows alternative ways of drawing a fingerprint

To test the validity of the model at this near completion stage, a formal research design was devised using a simulated patient to gather data to make and compare fingerprints.

SP Involvement in CEM Development

At two important points, simulated patient cases derived from real patient consultations (rpc) were used to confirm and develop thinking. Discussion regarding the make-up of the domains, for example, was spurred on by an informal research enquiry one evening at a local surgery. Three simulated patient cases were chosen from recordings of team members' consultations. The resulting SP cases were then filmed while the SPs consulted with pairs of Year 4 medical students, GP registrars, new GPs and two very experienced GPs. The recordings confirmed experiential differences and led to changes in the then domain list.

Later, once the indicative statements had been determined, the enquiry group felt it was necessary to re-focus on the question they started with, i.e. what is the nature of expert consulting? To achieve this, the enquiry team volunteered themselves to be recorded consulting with a challenging (rpc) patient (no consents required for this!). Two members subsequently fingerprinted all eight consultations recorded in group members' own consulting rooms. This further resulted in a comparison of two fingerprint scorers for the same case – introducing for the first time, the secondary question of fingerprint marking reliability.

Judith Anderson – a 'challenging' patient

Judith Anderson, a neatly dressed woman of 63, presents in a confused state clutching an empty packet of Nexium. She's uncertain why she made the appointment, but quickly describes the difficulty she has holding a knife, and asks: 'Why do I sit down when I come down the stairs?'. She wants to know what is happening to her and suggests a brain scan. She also wants to reduce her Diazepam dosage. Parkinson's disease has previously been suggested to explain her symptoms. Later in the consultation she asks, 'When I've had enough can I have nil by mouth?'

Mrs Anderson has a very long history of depression and agitation interspersed with other clinical conditions. Recently referred to a neurologist she has refused to change to the medication suggested. She says her husband does not share a life with her and she has no hugs.

'Difficulty' in this case occurs at three important levels – clinical, psychological and in her 'lifeworld' – each with significant complexity.

It was at this stage that a formal research enquiry was required if the Consultation Expertise Model was to be promoted in the public domain.

Research proposal

We proposed to record twenty general practitioners – ten experienced (more than ten years) and ten less experienced (three years or less) – consulting with the same rpc-simulated patient. The ten experienced doctors were all GP trainers. Each recording was then to be scored by four experienced GPs, thus producing a data collection of sixty-four fingerprints.

We were interested in discovering whether the indicative statement scoring system we devised does actually represent levels of expertise as shown in each of the eight domains. To achieve this, for each doctor consulting there would be four fingerprints to compare. In order to make this feasible a single simulated case was developed and shown to each of the twenty doctors.

Part of the research was intended to see whether distinct patterns of consulting can be distinguished between experienced and less experienced consultants. Thereby, to test the validity of the model and reliability of the fingerprint marking system. The reliability of simulated patients as a research resource was assumed from previous experience of using SPs for postgraduate learning and assessment.

Ethics Committee approval

Any research involving NHS employees or on NHS premises requires local Ethics Committee approval. For the use of a patient simulation, considerable thought was given by an ethics committee. This was because its presentation to a number of practices required consideration of the organisation and time required by doctors and practices. Organisation is highly time-consuming and is a major resource problem for any research project.

Ours was an unusual form of research. Committees are accustomed to considering proposals in terms of qualitative or quantitative research, which concerns either the handling of data or experimental therapies. A key point for us was enabling a committee to understand the process of obtaining the original rpc-consultation, because this can involve a de facto breach of confidentiality between the patient and the consulting doctor. Distinctively, ours was an educational rather than a medical research proposal.

Obtaining patient-doctor recordings requires adequate informed consent by the patient both before the consultation and afterwards. The committee required us to obtain the same level of informed consent from the consulting doctors. We also took the view that the recordings – although processed in an anonymised fashion – should remain in the ownership of the generating doctor.

Practical considerations

As a group of experienced GP educators, we'd been working with simulators for a long time and there was no question about their face validity. They'd been used with registrars in a training practice, with registrars in a group setting looking at particular skills and with poorly performing doctors. So we had a very clear idea that there was value in the simulations created through the Leicester rpc-method with its depth of patient representation. What we didn't know was whether that coupled with the model we'd derived could distinguish aspects of expertise or advanced consulting.

Most GPs are unfamiliar with the idea of simulated patients. We therefore needed a dialogue with interested doctors, to make sure they clearly understood what a simulation was and how they were expected to behave when it was presented to them. For example, because a simulation is contrived, some doctors may behave with it in a contrived manner.

To minimize this problem simulations were taken to the doctors' own practice so that the consultation could take place in their own consulting rooms, thus making it more possible for the doctor to behave as if it was one of his or her patients walking through the door. As important, the simulation had to represent a case the doctor would recognise as normal in daily practice. So the simulation was chosen from actual consultations made during routine practice. More important for research purposes, the case had to be sufficiently complex for consulting behaviour in each of the model's eight domains to be observed and scored by the independent scorers – though not so complex, particularly in psychological terms, that it would take hours to complete.

A suitable case

As we were interested in the behavioural differences of experienced compared with less experienced doctors, then clearly the more simplistic the case the less likelihood of behavioural differences being observed. We use the word 'challenge' for this. Challenge can be perceived in different ways. The first of these concerns the medical and clinical experience of the doctor. A case can be more complicated: if either its diagnosis is unclear or several diagnoses are running at the same time – so-called co-morbidities.

The second degree of challenge refers to whether there is something in the manner of the patient that challenges the doctor – such as an assertive or an aggressive person. Thirdly, there may be psychological issues such as depression that require particular forms of doctor behaviour even to engage the patient.

It happened by chance, but one reason for the choice of consultation was that a straight forward approach to any one of its problems was likely to have repercussions on other aspects. So, of necessity, compromises had to be identified and negotiated between the doctor and patient.

MALE	SUMMARY OF TREATMENT CARD	
Surname **HENDERSON**		Forename(s) *Margaret*
Address		
N.H.S. Number		Date of Birth Age **49 years**
Date		**Clinical Notes**
24 y ago		*Childbirth (M)*
22 y ago		*Childbirth (M)*
10 y ago		*TAH BSO – HRT Oestradiol Implant*

MALE	Surname		Forenames
	Address		
	N.H.S. Number		Date of Birth *49 years*
Date	*	Clinical Notes	
3 y ago		*SCIATICA*	
18 Months Ago		*Discussion of recurrent back problems Commenced on MELOXICAM, CO-CODAMOL*	
12 MONTHS AGO		*Chest Infection Rx Amoxicillin Smokes 40/day*	
10 Months ago		*Chest Infection Rx Cephalexin Given up smoking*	
9 Months ago		*Chest Infection Rx Erythromycin*	
6 m ago		*SOB. Lung Function Tests Consistent with COPD Refer to Chest Clinic*	
3 months ago		*Seen in Chest Clinic - COPD*	
2 Months ago		*In response to clinic letter started QVAR 100 2 bd Spiriva 15 mg daily Ipratroprium Inhaler pru Meloxicam 7.5 mg bd – Co-codamol 8/500 pru*	
		HRT implant review BP 130/80	

Patient – Margaret Henderson

The first thing I did was to take the recording of the original consultation between the GP and Margaret Henderson, not of course her real name – I'll never know the name of the real patient. I watched it from start to finish and transcribed everything exactly as it was said. I was also watching 'Margaret' for any little trait; she fiddles a lot with her glasses and with the beads round her neck. There's her general demeanour; her style of clothes; her make-up; her hair. I tried to take all that on board to ensure that I can replicate it as close as I can.

All her medical history was given to me in a format similar to the doctors' notes above, so I could see in chronological order when things happened in her life. When she had her children, any operations, any serious illnesses – it was all there. There was information about medication, any tests taken in places such as hospitals. The next stage, talking to the originating GP about the patient's backstory, was invaluable. I was able to find out things that do not come up on

the video but helped me build a bigger picture of Margaret Henderson as a person. At any one time I didn't know what direction a consultation would take – so this information gave me a better opportunity to remain consistent throughout, whatever the circumstances and whatever questions might be thrown at me. I discovered how many children she had, if her parents were still alive, what her home situation was like – her relationship with her husband, monetary situation and all that. Obviously, this was done with total confidentiality on my part. I didn't know and had never met this person, though at times I've felt I've become her.

When I do this role, I present with ongoing back pain that has not been successfully resolved over a period of two to three years. This is greatly complicated by another condition, chronic obstructive pulmonary disease, treated in hospital. If the doctor doesn't want to deal with the COPD, the implications are that a lot of cross-overs, such as mobility or lifestyle restrictions are not considered.
I'm very conscious not to provide anything for

the benefit of the doctor, i.e. by only responding to prompts. If a doctor approaches me in the right way to elicit certain information, that is fine. If the doctor fails to engage me, either with lack of warmth or rapport, then they will get absolutely nothing out of me.

As Margaret Henderson, I have complex medical issues, and if only the medical issues are dealt with but in a very empathetic and sympathetic way, I will be satisfied. However, I will have a much higher level of satisfaction if my home and work-world, my lifestyle, are entered into. Not in a brusque but in a sensitive manner. I'm quite a private person so the whole approach will be critical. I have two sons serving in Afghanistan, about whom I'm very worried. I wouldn't dream of mentioning them in a consultation unless my home life is touched upon. If asked, 'Who lives at home?' I will normally respond, 'Just me and my husband now'. if the 'now' is picked up I may volunteer that both sons are in the army. That opens up a whole new area of my worries and concerns. What I might say about my husband, bearing in mind my back problems, is that I've felt it necessary to have a cleaner. He disapproves, strongly disapproves. If the doctor takes that up and explores our relationship, as it relates to my medical condition, they'll get more information – about the fact that we only have one family car so I have to spend hours on end at a bus stop, which I resent. It is information that helps them further the medical outcome though they are not asking medical questions, just getting to know me as a person.

I am well aware that I must present the same patient challenge in every consultation. We know from other work that we have to 'cleanse', to present anew from consultation to consultation. Whatever questions are thrown at me, I respond as I think my character would, according to the background information. Given the amount going on in Margaret Henderson's life, together with such clear personality parameters (from the video), it's fairly easy to retain consistency.

Sometimes I do get a feeling, 'is this going to be like a play acting experience?' But within a short period of time, every doctor I encounter treats me as a real patient. Any reservations are soon dissipated. I feel that I'm treated throughout as a patient.

The Margaret Henderson case presents a challenge for proficient to expert doctors at three levels:

1. Clinical – COPD +chronic backache
2. Psychological – the condition is causing disturbance to the marital relationship
3. Personal – effects on conditions at work, fears about the safety of her sons and the lack of sympathy shown by her husband

Securing the evidence

The consultations were recorded with twenty doctors of varying experience, and this meant journeying with the SP to practices across the East Midlands over a period of three weeks. All participating doctors were aware of the manner of case development and the need to consider the case as part of an ordinary working day. On arrival, the camera was installed while the SP waited to be called and the doctor was given basic rules of procedure:

- The 'patient' can be examined
- Assume that there are no other patients in the waiting room or pressures such as ten minute consultation routines.

Analysing the evidence

Two of the recordings were used to induct and moderate the four doctor scorers into the practice of making case-fingerprints with sufficient consistency to be sent to the external evaluator. The scorers were doctors who had not previously been in contact with the CEM model.

Fortunately, the four doctors proved to be adept learners and the moderation discussions led to comparable marking practice. The four then spent two days at separate TV screens making fingerprints of the sixteen recordings. No comment was made by scorers regarding the variation of simulated patient challenge during this intense and detailed process – a significant omission.

Research Findings

The data sent to the external evaluator provided sufficient validity correlation between domains and domain descriptions to support the fingerprinting process. The evidence also indicated marking process reliability. More interesting perhaps is the fact that five GP trainers and three new doctors were placed in the top eight ranking. A finding that conflicts with the assumption that all experienced trainers will consult at a higher level than newcomers.

Using SPs for research

The project highlighted a set of facilitation factors necessary for the successful use of a simulated patient as the sole resource for data collection:

* **The choice of an experienced SP to represent a patient case of suitable challenge is of paramount importance, as are supporting details such as case notes and examination cards, where applicable.**
* Attention is needed to ensure that all those likely to be directly concerned are familiar with simulated patient practice.
* Similar thought should be given to Ethics Committee applications and committee members' familiarity with SPs.
* All the above involve detailed organisational attention, as do the minutiae of the research programme and its application.

On reflection, given our previous use of SPs both for assessment and learning, we were confident that the simulator and case chosen would serve the research purpose well. What we didn't do was either prepare contingency plans for things going wrong or establish a means to verify the standardisation of the challenge. If our findings became subject to serious questioning on the basis of variable SP challenge, our fallback position would have been the apparent satisfaction of experienced GP scorers. But, we did not think to collect evidence on that score, an important omission concerning the integrity of the evidence.

Conclusion

This enquiry was structured around a simulated patient as a data generating resource. Experienced SPs can present as near reality patients – or for that matter as doctors, nurses or relatives – and can not only present a consistent challenge, but also respond uniquely at each encounter. This highlights their potential usefulness as a research tool. In the above case, simulation artifice was widely understood and its use agreed. Studies have been conducted and published using SPs as proxy or 'undercover' patients, usually to assess the quality of GP consulting practice. Often this is with prior agreement, but secret filming by SPs has been undertaken to expose poor practice – an uneasy situation for the SPs involved. Furthermore, while the potential to use SPs in this standardized manner may be advantageous for certain kinds of research, the above sample of twenty consistent contacts may be about the limit for one simulated case – human simulators do have human limitations.

Dr Adrian French was at the time a practicing GP and VTS Course Organiser (now called Programme Directors). Carolyn Oldershaw is a well experienced SP who produces audio book recordings and is a 'voiceover' artist.

Seven

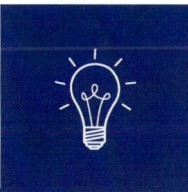

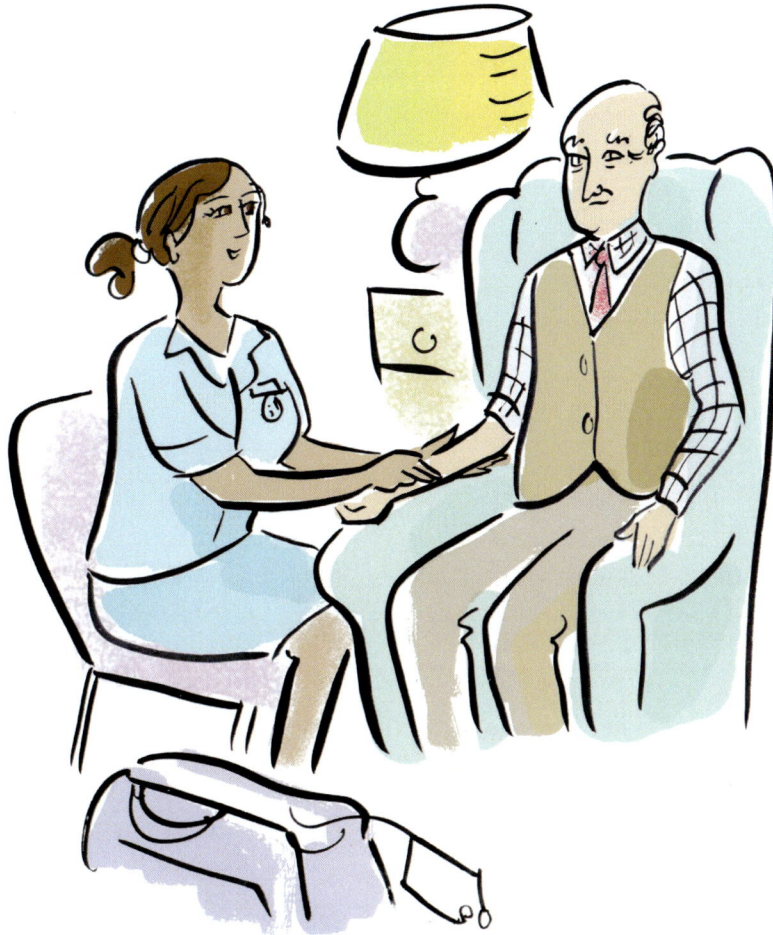

Advance Care Planning Workshop for Community Nurses

Interview with Carole Tallon

The interview is in response to questions from a simulated patient who had been facilitated by Carole Tallon and others during the experiential part of the Advance Care Planning course

How did this course on advance care planning come about?

Within Coventry and Warwickshire, Dr Dan Munday – lecturer at the University of Warwick and a consultant in palliative medicine in Coventry – is a lead on the Health Innovations Education Cluster Project (HIEC) for training in End of Life Care. One of the things Dan is working on is the promotion of advance care planning. In terms of the required documentation, we decided to develop it from a national model. Dan got a group of us together, including Dr Jo Poultney who is the educational lead. The group largely consisted of local palliative care consultants. All the Trusts and the independent Hospice were involved. Everybody in our locality signed up to it. HIEC provided us with a two-year funding stream so that we could devise the documentation and roll it out to train local healthcare professionals. This involved: how to use the documentation; how to present it to patients and fill it in with them; and how to communicate the contents to other health workers and agencies. There is also an action research element so we can evolve the programme.

In terms of the national end-of-life care programme there is a politically driven agenda to find people's preferences, with a large emphasis on preferred place of death. The reasons behind this are that hospital care is costly and there is an imperative to reduce unnecessary admissions. Also, although more people die in hospital than at home, surveys suggest that the majority (but not all) would like to die at home. The Preferred Priorities for Care documents and the Advance Decision to Refuse Treatment document together form an Advance Care Plan. There is a national document but it is being customised for use in some localities.

To what extent are you under pressure because it is cheaper if people don't die in hospital?

We sense that the Government would like us to introduce advance care planning in order to promote people dying at home. It is easy to see that hospital care is expensive, but if the patient needs more care at home than they are currently receiving, then this may be cheaper but may not serve the patient's needs. From our professional experience, we know that people may say they want to die at home but that is not the whole story – in an ideal world they might like to die at home but when circumstances find them left alone or their partner can't cope, they get frightened and/or their symptoms become too distressing to manage. Maybe there isn't enough support in the community from agencies such as district nursing and care services. We are aware that the advance care planning needs to establish what the patients' preferences are with reassurance that the patient can change his or her mind at any time. We also need to communicate to patients that this isn't about choosing from a menu, and that a stated preference does not guarantee that

outcome because of multiple variables, such as a spouse not being able to cope.
The Advance Care Planning document needs to be understood as a living dynamic on-going discussion. Though we must be mindful that there are some legal aspects, such as Advance Decision to Refuse Treatment.

This sounds like a very sophisticated project given the various professional people involved?

You're absolutely right. It is much more complicated than it looks on the surface. The national initiative (EOLC strategy), in their algorithm of what happens during the last year of life, suggests that at some stage you have the conversation with the patient. Preferences and circumstances change – it needs to be an on-going conversation.

What do you see as the context of the one-day training?

The message we hope will be gained is that this is a patient-focused approach – to find out what the patient understands. So we expect the health care professionals will have consulted with other professionals who've agreed that the time has come to initiate a conversation about the end of life. A district nurse is unlikely to have that conversation without discussing it with a GP. Within the pack there are guidelines to say who it gets communicated to. That's all part of the training day. Anybody who comes into contact with a patient might end up having the conversation. A patient may open up to a health care assistant while having a bath, but at this stage we are not opening up the training to health care assistants, so they can't fill in the forms. We would hope that the health care assistant would pass on the information. By and large, the people coming on the training are likely to be in the forefront of care and likely to be making decisions. They are people who have been dealing with these patients for a number of years. The training day is a way of formalising the kind of conversations they are probably having anyway. It's giving the health care professional permission to have this conversation, and to enable or at least facilitate the patient's desired outcomes.

When you set about designing the day, how did you decide what to do?

We looked at the amount of information we needed to give. We tweaked it a little bit and made a joint decision on the need for half a day of experiential learning. The morning session is interactive so that people have the opportunity to put their points across. It's made clear that their professional duty is to go away and read the pack. Our own professional knowledge of learning made it essential to put in an experiential part. We didn't want people to go away feeling that they had been talked at but not having plumbed the depths of their own knowledge and experience.

That sounds like the process of awareness, understanding and application?

We are all palliative care doctors so all our training has been of doing it.
Some of us have been trained as GPs, so we all have facilitator experience and have been specialty trainers.

What are the main parts of the course?

In the morning there is an introduction to advance care planning, its purpose and importance. We show them the evidence, for example, that people who are able to plan are less likely to suffer from anxiety and depression. We go through the documentation and the ethics (people do struggle as to whether it's even ethical to bring up the subject). We look at autonomy and where choice, justice and the utilisation of resources are involved. We also look at beneficence and non-maleficence.

There is a concentration on ethics while we are looking at the actual document. We talk about prognostication for various kinds of diseases. We remind them that it's also about whether the patient wants to talk about this. We tell them that they can practise in the afternoon.

Then we show them a short film. It is a cartoon about a little old lady who is resuscitated by a well-meaning (but misguided and uninformed medical team) – a struggle between the grim reaper and the doctor.

Then we have lunch.

In the afternoon there are two or three groups of about ten. In each group there's a facilitator, a co-facilitator and a simulated patient who presents three scenarios of the type of patient likely to be encountered. The characters are fictitious but based on real-life cases.

Scenario One – George Y

Mr George Y is a 66 year old man with end-stage Parkinson's disease who lives at home with his wife. He has progressive reduced mobility and slowing of speech. He has recently been seen as an outpatient by his neurologist who felt he was receiving maximum therapy for his Parkinson's disease and could be offered no further treatment. He has recently been discharged from hospital where he was admitted with a chest infection and he has clearly deteriorated further, needing carers several times a day and a hoist for transfers. He was in the acute hospital for three weeks which his wife reports he found quite distressing at times.

Facilitator and Simulated Patient notes

Mr Y is aware that his condition is deteriorating and knows he has reached the limit of his Parkinson's medication. He is surprised by the discussion regarding advance care planning and being able to record his wishes as it is

not something he is familiar with. He is quite willing to participate in the discussion and volunteers without prompting that he does not want to be brought back to life if his heart stops. He needs direction regards other aspects of his care.

His preferred place of care is home.

He would only want other treatment that would warrant transfer to hospital if it would improve his quality of life (e.g. antibiotics, artificial feeding and I.V fluids)

We want the SP to be Mr Y so the facilitator can work with each group member through him to explore how best to elicit his thoughts and feelings about the future.

Scenarios Two and Three are used to introduce other concepts in the pack which are commonly brought up by patients: 'living wills'; dying with dignity; the patient who doesn't have a preference about where to die. Dealing with such specifics helps to improve delegates' skills. Patients may not have thought about who is going to take care of them. We know health workers may make a lot of assumptions. Going back to the political agenda, some may now feel their remit is to persuade people to die at home, and may feel that is what they have to get the patient to sign up to. So the second scenario is to create a realisation that the patient may want something different – much of the day is about breaking down assumptions.

The third scenario is to show them that the patient may not want to talk about this at all. We put that in to make sure they don't go away thinking 'We talked about this wonderful documentation set and skills to elicit the information so we can now go out and do it'. They need to go away with the message that it's OK not to do it, if the patient doesn't want to. It's not about achieving a 100% target.

I'm intrigued to know how you regard facilitating with simulated patients. I've observed you keeping a tighter rein than most?

I do have my own style. But I've been on the 3 day National "Connect" – Advanced Communication Skills Training course where, on the first day, the SP is there for a group scenario. You can spend lunch time with the SP and talk about the delegates' skill levels. You can set it up with the simulator and that is what I am used to doing. With the Advance Care Planning course we have a very limited time with ten delegates, each of whom only sits in the chair once. Therefore, we have to make sure that everyone has a meaningful, affirming, safe experience. There is a massive responsibility on both the SP and the facilitator. These scenarios are very straight forward, only open to a little interpretation. Our learning objectives are that the delegate will elicit the patient's agenda. Do they know that they are dying? Have they got any preferences? What are the things they don't want to happen? How do they feel about filling in a form? Filling in the form itself within the training session was never part of the plan. The objective is that they will be confident enough to elicit the patient's ideas, concerns and expectations and be able to respond to their emotions – their ICEE.

I have a frustration that, as a group, we have not made our objectives clear regarding communication skills, despite the fact that achieving the above depends upon them. Opportunities to highlight these skills may occur but only on an opportune basis as there is no time to focus on them. It's a big remit in a mixed ability group! That said, we do distribute a communication advice sheet to be read during or after the activity. It is something we will work on going forward.

Going back to the question of facilitation, firstly I think the facilitator has to be personable and should make it clear at the start that they are not an expert. They are there to facilitate the learning of everyone in the room. Nevertheless, as facilitator, you are in charge and you have to be quite directive within the ground rules. We do go through them to establish safety – specifically that it's OK to leave the room (if someone gets upset). You can lighten the atmosphere – it's difficult to harm an SP! I also remind them that it's not role play – they tend to be scared of role play. They must be themselves and not act a role.

I try to establish what we will be doing in each next little section, e.g.

'I am now going to find out what the patient knows about his illness'.

If you are not directive about that and they go beyond that contract, you have to stop it. The learning objective, in this case, is learning what the patient knows. I make it clear that I will stop them if there is a learning point or if they go off track. Or, if they get stuck, they can stop by going 'time out'.

Feedback?

We are accustomed to using Pendleton's rules to give one another feedback. First we look at all the positives, and then the constructive feedback will be about how it might have been done differently. Sometimes, they start by saying, 'Oh, I shouldn't have done such and such'. We stop them and say, 'Hang on. Remember we said we'd do what went well first'. By facilitating the feedback properly like this, you are reinforcing the good in what everybody does. Getting the feedback well facilitated is probably more than 50% of the good work. One hopes they are practising empathetically and so showing empathy is emphasised and applauded. The good thing about having the delegates observe each other is that they all get some learning from watching those in the chair.

There's a problem for us in that we get excellent feedback from the delegates. That de-motivates us for changing and improving it. I am always a little sceptical about evaluations. Have we set them up not to be specific enough? Are they tired at the end of the day when they fill it in and so do not have the energy to give constructive comments?

From the simulator's point of view.

I can remember the first time I was George Y. All those who occupied the chair created a rapport of some kind but I couldn't understand why they wouldn't come clean and say what it was they wanted from me, i.e. what is this care plan you are talking about? I'm now clear that your agenda is only to concentrate on the first stage with George, i.e. preparing the ground for a care plan. Only the facilitator can determine this learning boundary.

Given that Stan, in scenario three, 'doesn't want to talk about the future', having only read the scenario, I reacted very quickly the first time I did it. This was because I saw Stan as being too upset, even angry, at the oncologists' information that there was no further treatment. So, I only communicated non-verbally. I now understand that it doesn't matter which way I react as long as it leads to the person in the chair realising that this is not the time to delve into my feelings.

Is there an afterthought?

Amongst ourselves we need to be clearer on the specifics of our learning objectives, so we can work better with the SPs. That means keeping it fairly straightforward. This is about the basic communication skills required to have end-of-life care discussions. If health workers have well-thought-out discussions with patients, they can then fill in the documentation that enables them to network and communicate with all the agencies. In that way their patients' preferences are more likely to be met.

Dr Carole Tallon is Director of the Coventry Myton Hospice

Eight

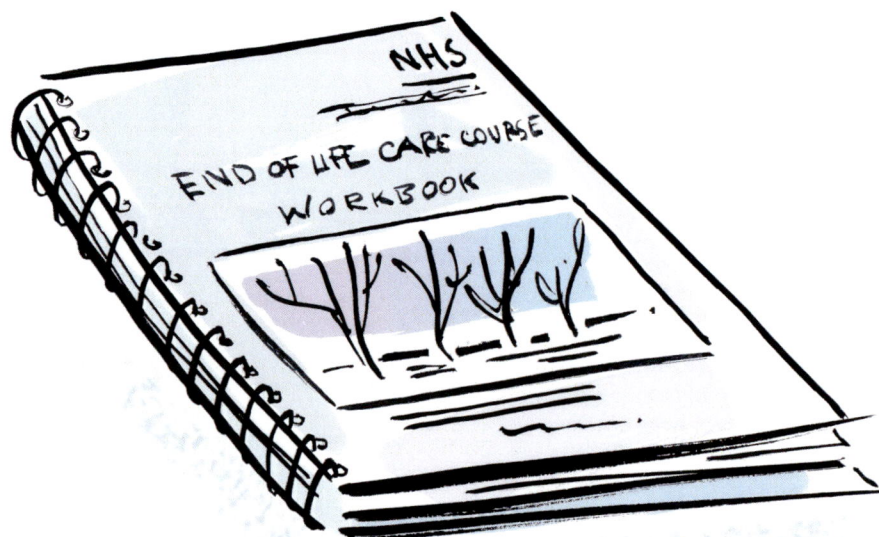

End of Life Care Course for GP Specialty Registrars

Stuart Holloway

Origins

The End of Life Care Course was designed in response to a Deanery directive to develop end of life care training for GP speciality registrars (GPRs) before they enter practice following their certification of completion of training. I was asked to lead on the development of a course that could be replicated across the Deanery. Initially I endeavoured to seek out the learning needs of GP registrars through the organisation of a questionnaire survey of ST3 GP registrars, programme directors, district nurses, and palliative care consultants across the East Midlands Deanery. The findings were utilised in the development of the course curriculum and template for an end of life care course that could be used by different GP training programmes across the East Midlands. The template permitted flexibility for programmes

to run courses according to local need and the course subsequently ran across all of these programmes. I have remained responsible for the course provided for registrars on the Derby programme – a two day course originally offered to GP registrars in their third year. Feedback has indicated that the skills and mindset acquired on the course would be more beneficial if it is run a year earlier. This year (2013) second and third year GP registrars have attended the course, as a transitional arrangement.

A significant portion of the course is devoted to developing communication skills, since it is clear that such skills are essential for providing quality care. Small group work with simulated patients is central to the success of the course and takes up a significant proportion of the first day.

The clinical scenarios, written especially, are based on real end of life events witnessed in general practice. They involve patients and family members. There is added value in that the more sensitive, interpersonal skills practised on the course can be used more generally.

Objectives

There are two principal learning objectives. The first is to ensure that the GP registrars enhance their ability to manage end of life care. The second is to develop and enhance their communication skills, such that they learn to adapt effectively to clinical circumstances. A number of registrars struggle with communication skills, particularly with regard to being patient-centred, so the course is designed to enhance these skills in the context of current provision in palliative and cancer care, district nurse and Macmillan nurse provision and other relevant ethical and legal issues. Furthermore, throughout the two days, we are able to raise levels of understanding and knowledge of the available support agencies.

There are existing frameworks to support end of life care in the revised GP Training Curriculum (Chapter 12 deals with cancer and palliative care needs) and in the Gold Standards Framework for Palliative Care. The course enables registrars to become aware of, absorb and apply many of these recommendations.

Course sessions relate not just to communication skills, but to other aspects of end of life care management such as wills and advanced directives, benefits and social care, therapeutics in palliative care, palliative care emergencies, cancer prevalence and screening, the Quality and Outcomes Framework, two week referral guidelines, significant event analysis, religious and cultural beliefs, and ethics. Much of this involves crossing professional boundaries, all of which is necessary if the approach is to be holistic, and the teaching provision is truly multi-professional. In the session on cultural beliefs for example, the hospital chaplain explains how beliefs across the world influence how death is managed.

Information and Discussion Sessions

Gold Standard Framework

Role of Macmillan Nurses

Therapeutics in Palliative care

Wills & Advanced Directives

Quality Outcomes Framework

Cancer Prevalence and Screening

Ethics in Palliative Care

Cultural Beliefs

The Simulated Patient Sessions

The simulated patient sessions occupy a significant part of the course. There are eight written scenarios, all of which involve a short life expectancy ranging from hours to, at most, a few weeks. Group numbers are small enough for each registrar to deal with at least one case and observe three others; altogether these sessions can be emotionally draining.

Some registrars are naturally competent in communication skills. Some require quite a lot of input. Uppermost in my mind is making sure, when such cases occur, that these registrars choose an appropriate environment, i.e. have some situational awareness; that they use open questions, develop effective listening skills and become more comfortable in discussing and explaining prognoses and future management plans with palliative care patients and their relatives, sharing decision making with both groups. Explaining what might happen clinically requires knowledge, empathy and skill. We encourage the GPRs to look out for cues and as they develop their skills, they will spend a lot of time prioritising and filtering cues and deciding how to respond. Simulators help with this because they feed back which cues should prompt a response. Simulated patients stay in role for the duration of the consultation but are frequently asked for feedback out of role. We know from past experience that these simulated patients present as authentic patients. They are able to adapt their responses rapidly and effectively to the needs of the registrar and, if called upon, can present in a different state of mind; for example, they can change the mood of the patient to anger or grief.

It is clear from observing sessions that end of life scenarios demand behaviours that may be experienced infrequently in daily GP consultations:

The two extracts below may seem difficult to follow. Both occur later in the consultation when the patient feels free to express their innermost feelings. They talk as they think!

How long have I got and what will happen?

The patient is a woman in her eighties with a cardiac problem who has called the doctor for a home visit because she got so short of breath last night.

Dr	Do you have any idea of what's going on with your heart – your breathing?
Pt	Not much you can do – I couldn't breathe – thought I'd had it.
Dr	Can stop you feeling breathless [pause]
Pt	Is this it? I need to know. I'm worried about Eric.
Dr	Would you like me to be honest?
Pt	Scary isn't it?
Dr	Couple of options – fluid building up – hospital …

Pt	Not under any circumstances – not leaving Eric.
Dr	You don't have very long – I'd say less than a day.
Pt	Thank you, I thought that might be the case. Better to know. Will you look after him? He won't manage, you know. Do I just go to sleep – what happens?

Time Out

Time was spent in the group feedback discussing how to explain what might happen, bearing in mind that we can only make a reasonable prediction if the patient agrees to palliative therapeutic care – an undercurrent of the extract.

How to help?

This next extract is from a surgery-based consultation with a 30 year old married woman with two children. Surgery has followed a delayed diagnosis of breast cancer, which in turn was followed by protracted chemotherapy. She has metastatic disease and has been informed no further treatment is possible.

Dr	Shall we start by talking about the pain?
Pt	I'm taking the tablets but the pain is worse.
Dr	Do you have ideas about what's best to do?
Pt	Morphine – I'm struggling to go to the toilet.
Dr	Maybe take the morphine in a different way. [long pause]
Pt	Do they all have similar side-effects – it's feeling sick and having no energy.
Dr	How are you coping at home?
Pt	I want to see my kids – I don't want to spend my last times not talking to them – I can talk to them but they don't want to hear it.
Dr	How would you feel if we talked to the family?

Pt   I feel I ought to get things sorted – write my will. I feel it's all changing so quickly – how can I make sure they will be all right?

Dr   Have you seen any of the nurses?

Pt   Cross bridges when we come to them – can't get up and go to the kitchen easily. I just want to change a few things.

Time Out

A common feedback factor in both extracts was the demeanour of the doctors; both leaned forward with unwavering empathic eye contact and spoke in warm, quiet, tones with invitational pauses. The patients' feelings were not impeded by the doctors' concerns. 'I didn't feel you had an agenda; it felt natural and organic', was one patient's feedback to the doctor.

Facilitation

Group facilitators must have an interest in palliative care and be able to run a small group of around 4 to 5 GP registrars. They need to identify registrars who are less willing to take part in the scenarios and enable their engagement in the process. They need to be able to assist the registrars with determining how well they have done and what improvements they can make as well as facilitating feedback from the other registrars in a positive and constructive manner. They need to be able to work alongside the simulator and have an understanding as to how the simulators work. They may have palliative care skills but in these sessions the focus is very much on communication as opposed to the detail of therapeutics and so on.

In reality, for an individual GP, the number of palliative care patients at any one time will be small; however, they are a very important group who often need assistance and management decisions made at short notice, and the GP needs to know how to handle that.

The scenarios focus on a range of problems, maybe an urgent home visit late on Friday night or one with a relative expressing concern about the patient's care. As will be seen from the illustrations above, dealing with such cases demands special skills. Although facilitators may have palliative care experience, given that these are active learning episodes, they should hold back on giving personal advice – with exceptions! I'll give you an example of that from my own experience: the use of syringe drivers features in the course but GPs may use them infrequently. When the need does arise, the GP may not feel certain about which drugs to combine, or how to make opiate conversions accurately. Personally, I ring the pharmacist every time and I advise registrars to do the same. Last thing on a Friday night they may well have forgotten what they were taught on the course.

Outcomes

The course is supported by a comprehensive workbook and virtual learning programme. We ask for feedback every year but this is limited to feelings about the course, not about how registrars will use what they have learnt. Their feedback suggests that registrars gain a lot from the course and they mention the communication skills in particular. Realistically, a GP with a list size of 1800 patients may have only 2 to 3 patients at any one time in a terminal state. To that you may add up to 10 patients being treated palliatively: those who are expected to die within 12 months. Though small in number, they require specialised clinical expertise.

Dr Stuart Holloway is a practicing General Practitioner, GP Trainer, GP Appraiser, and Programme Director at the Derby GP Speciality Training Programme.

Nine

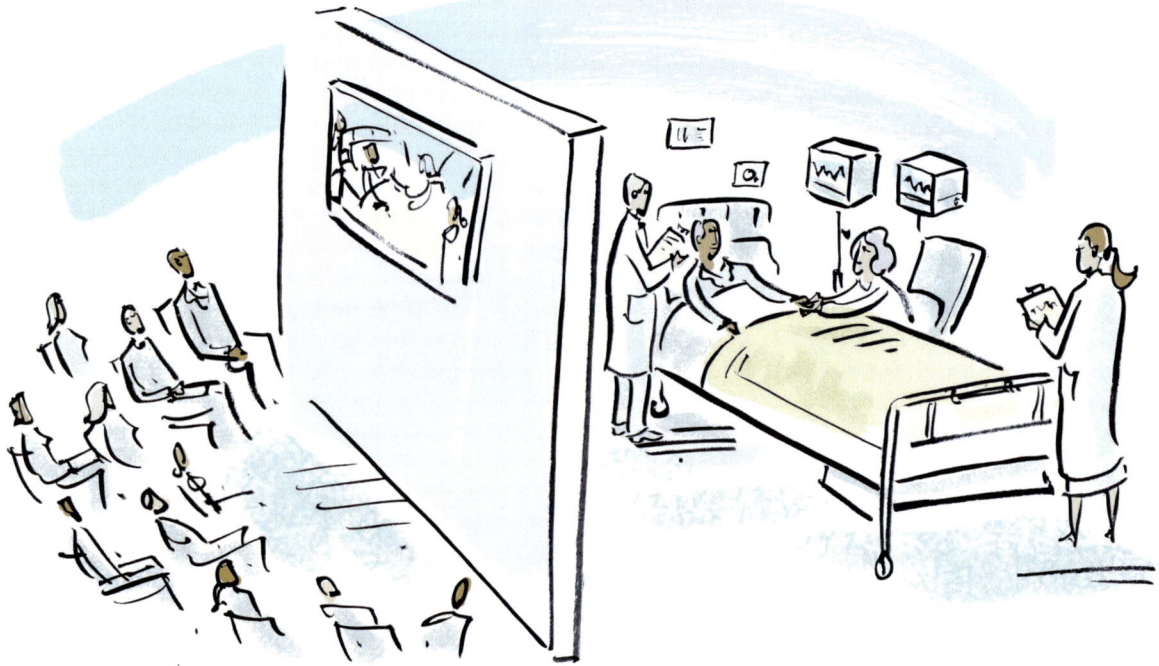

Working with a High-Tech 'Simulated Patient'

Andy Buttery

Place of work

The simulation room, known in the UK by most users, as the 'sim' room, is part of the Trent Simulation and Clinical Skills Centre (TS&CSC), located in the Medical Education Centre at the Queens Medical Centre, Nottingham University NHS Hospitals Trust. Adjacent to it are rooms containing high-tech machines used for endoscopy training and part-task artificial body parts. The Centre is designed to serve the clinical training needs of hospital staff, medical students and health professionals such as dentists. The initiative to build, as I see it, resulted from the happy coincidence of drug company funding in conjunction with the drive and vision of Dr Bryn Baxendale (Centre Director). His hands-on experience gained from simulation training

with anaesthetists, plus support from the Dean of the (then) Trent-Multi Professional Deanery, guaranteed a building fit for purpose.

The TS&CSC began operating with an exclusive secondary care, in-house perspective – the high-tech end of the simulation spectrum. This changed in 2009 with the adoption of a 30-plus team of simulated patients accustomed to working in a variety of off-site primary care situations – at the 'live', not even low-tech end of the spectrum.

The 'sim' room

Imagine you're in the corridor of a building adjacent to a major hospital. To your left and right are doors and ahead is another door. Go first left and you'll find yourself in a space like the control room of a television studio. In front is a wide shelf with microphone, monitors, telephones and other equipment. Look through the one-way glass wall and you'll see a hospital bed surrounded by everything needed for clinical care. There are chairs for visitors and a telephone. On the bed is a plastic patient, a manikin, capable of simulating most bodily functions. Hardly visible are television cameras. Exiting into the corridor you can enter the third room – the seminar-viewing room. Here you'll find a circle of chairs, a whiteboard, a large screen monitor and speakers relaying everything that goes on in the 'sim' room. There is capability to show activity both in real-time and recorded time.

The patient is a dummy, but this dummy can speak and respond as a person. Its voice has the immediacy of any human's; it's the voice of whoever is using the microphone, be it a man or a woman. The dummy has a pulse, blood pressure, heart and lung sounds, and fluids – most dramatically, blood. The chest moves with breath, the eyes blink and the pupils contract. With this technology in a complete clinical environment it becomes possible to simulate a multiplicity of acute clinical conditions, illustrating what might happen on a typical day in hospital.

Groups engaged in simulation training

Groups regularly booked for training range from anaesthetists to school students who visit with a view to considering potential careers in health work. Putting aside occasional courses such as Patient Safety in Theatre Teams, there is an annual rotation of courses for:

- Final year medical students
- Foundation years 1 & 2 (F1-F2)
- Core Medical Training (CMT 1/2)
- Managing Medical Emergencies for Dental Practices
- Dental Foundation Year trainees

A typical simulation training day

The participants are a group of eight F1 doctors, some of whom may have previous experience of working in the 'sim' room as final year medical students. The day is structured in three stages.

Stage One - *Briefing*

First we introduce the ground rules of simulation training in a 'safe learning environment' and discuss video recording and debriefing. Then we introduce the 'sim' room and the manikin, paying finickety attention to detail: every word is considered. We have learnt from a classic error we first made with medical students, one of whom had an adrenalin syringe in hand and was about to administer the drug into a vein and thereby probably harm the patient. Moments like this are what simulation learning is all about. While this concerns clinical knowledge, it also raises behavioural issues around team working and patient safety – how might the team avoid this error (or one like it) in future? Furthermore, this could be an example of how we call up memory – the candidates have arrived expecting to resuscitate a manikin – and adrenaline is given directly into the vein during resuscitation attempts. But the layered golden learning opportunity is completely lost if we haven't shown the group how to give the manikin an intra-muscular injection. The manikin has pads on its shoulders for this purpose. If we forget to mention it in the induction, we have to inform them mid action and undermine the 'reality' of the scenario.

In the viewing room there are eight F1 doctors briefed for action throughout the day. Both individually and in small teams, they will confront a series of different scenarios chosen to elicit a range of clinical and behavioural learning points. Those not engaged in the scenario will be able to see and hear what happens in the seminar-viewing room where they may often be required to record observations. I will usually be in the control room with other faculty team members and technicians. By the side of the patient there will be ECG, BP, and blood-oxygenation data on the monitor. A nurse will be in attendance.

Stage Two – *Action*

To create a typical case, the patient on a surgical ward is young and fit but needs an operation for appendicitis. He has a fluid drip with antibiotics running into an arm cannula. One or both of the doctors have been asked 'to see Mr Cummings with appendicitis who is complaining of being short of breath'. The doctors enter the ward and confirm that the patient is short of breath and has low oxygen levels. They give him oxygen but his BP is falling, so they give him some fluids. Gradually they build up a picture that this patient is having an anaphylactic reaction to something and they commence the clinical procedure, which is to give intra-muscular adrenaline (IMA).

Stage Three – *Debriefing*

The actual performance is both predictable and unique. It falls within the normal distribution bell-curve of expected clinical competence, and it is the real behavior of a unique group of individuals living through an actual experience (albeit a simulation). For example, the moment when the antibiotics are noticed varies from 'very soon' to 'never'. When the scenario is over we might say, 'What was causing the allergic reaction?' To which they may reply, 'I don't know'. This can be one of those light-bulb learning moments. I've often felt inclined to comment, 'You wouldn't have believed me if I'd said earlier: you will be called to see a patient on a ward with a drip running, who is having an anaphylactic reaction, but you will not check what is in the drip'. If they are stressed as they step into the ward or as they struggle to complete clinical tasks, they can lose the overview. Whether their stress results from crisis with the patient or from the fact that they are being observed and filmed, I don't care, and I'm usually quite happy to accept their own opinion on the matter, providing they accept in return that they will be equally, if not more stressed, for different reasons at work. The lessons about behaviour are valid and should be transferrable into practice.

How we open the debrief presents us with an intuitive puzzle – how best to facilitate discussion? Often it will be, 'Tell us about the patient you met…' or 'How did you feel when ….?' With the help of selected recordings we'll prompt them to discuss what happened. We'll sit and listen as they progress from description, to extracting reasons, to reflecting on what they have done. We intervene to support them in identifying strategies to improve performance. We might interrupt with questions such as, 'If that was your plan, why didn't you share it with the patient or the rest of the team?'

Video clips enable us to focus on the candidate. For example, at worst, s/he may say to the patient 'How are you doing today Mr Jones? I'm Dr Smith, I'm here to look after you'. And Mr Jones says 'I've had me leg off you know'. To which somewhat farcically but nonetheless typically, the response might be, 'Um yes, airways OK?' You show them the clip and say 'How were your communication skills there?' Mention the word 'communication' and the response may be along the lines of, 'Well we've done communication skills!' But now they've applied their theoretical learning in context, do they really understand what, for instance, 'active listening' requires in real patient contact? Or do they only know the buzz words? Watching themselves can be cathartic! At the same time of course, it opens up a learning opportunity for us.

Making it happen

Simulation for clinical learning covers a wide range of activity. At one extreme there are those who work intermittently with small groups using SPs to focus on patient-doctor communication. At the other, there are the solitary learners who practise surgical procedures on high-tech machines. In between are those who use part-task trainers in groups guided by facilitators. In the 'sim' room, what happens involves clinical activity, interpersonal communication and group learning. Each session involves a faculty team of four or five people. Furthermore, this is done on average four days out of five. As a consequence, organization and facilitation become one and the same thing.

Starting point – *the first time with a real patient won't be your first time*

If simulation here only achieves one thing, it's that for candidates unaccustomed to real responsibility on a ward, meeting a problem for the first time won't really feel like the first time if it's already been encountered during a simulation exercise. Contradictory perhaps, but if doctors have anxieties about starting work they can come here and see what they may do in a safe environment, free from worries about harming patients. And they can experience how they will perform in relation to their peers, who may also be worried about self-image. From that point on we need to be wary of what we do. We can and do, for instance, flatten 'sim' experience for some and enhance it for others. To explain:

In the 'sim' room we have the luxury of playing with time. We can slow down the clock, slow down the deterioration of the patient or jump forward in time; if that's what we need to do. Learners are not interacting with a text book, with a cipher that is always the same – they are interacting with a ward nurse who will react differently if the participant smiles at them and says 'Can you help me with this chap, I think he is really sick'. There are all sorts of things going on. What that might lead to if we have a candidate who is clinically very good, and performing quite well is that we'll make the patient get sick very quickly. The staff will be friendly but won't feel they need to be particularly supportive and everything will be stacked against that good candidate demonstrating a slick performance – but stacked in favour of learning as much as possible. There are subtleties in the interactions

of the learners: how they are comparing themselves to each other, the difference between what they say about a performance whilst observing it and what they actually feed back to the participant in the debrief. And of course they all take part in each stage so they know what is happening and must wonder what has been left unsaid. The danger is that learners leave with inappropriate self-belief or unrealistic ideas of consequence. The faculty training team have to guard and guide against this.

Some challenge may be deliberate on our part, or 'en passant', as it happens in and around what we are trying to achieve with the scenario. For the struggling candidate: the patient will not deteriorate so quickly; the staff will offer suggestions; the phone call from the senior (advice can be called for from the telephone by the bed) will be more helpful, so the candidate will be buoyed up (it's us on the phone). Our defence for such engineering is that we provide a learning opportunity not an assessment. This illustrates a different level of facilitation from, say the excellent Advanced Life Support (ALS) course with its measurement of knowledge and skills, where you have to clear a competence hurdle to get a certificate irrespective of whether you do a triple somersault over the hurdle or not. However, we aim to provide our learners with the opportunity, one day, to be triple somersaulters. Though rarely made explicit, we like to think professionalism and excellence underpin the agenda of a good simulation course. A good performance no longer just means 'You've passed'. Now it means 'Let's take that apart and discover (for everyone) the behaviour that made it so good.'

It's our intention to provide the conditions to experience the maximum number of learning opportunities. We hope this is the case for all those who come through simulation training, including those who vicariously enjoy it as peer observers. So our struggling candidate has an easier time and will come through buoyed up.

Our brilliant candidate will come out having had a reasonably good time, unaware of being streets ahead, because we've flattened their performance. Next year they may be the one to forget to check the drip – they are still human. We are not about assessing or ranking them, we are about providing learning opportunities.

A discrete learning issue – *handover*

Handover from one clinician to another occurs day and night in hospital, and it presents an opportunity and a risk. The opportunity is to respond in the moment, to make sure everything is in hand by insisting on meticulous attention to detail. The risk is an incomplete and potentially dangerous handover. In the simulation centre the facilitator can bring other people in to highlight this essential skill. We can have one learner sitting in isolation so they know nothing about the situation they walk into. Or, you can take a learner out of the observation room, where, although they've watched on the screen, they don't know what's in the heads of people round the bed. They must still get a handover – and in one sense they are up to speed – but they must know what's in other people's heads.

Added complexity – *the presence of relatives*

In recent years we've introduced 'live' simulators (SPs) into the scenarios as patients, relatives and occasionally as problem staff members. We've learnt a lot about how best to use them and they are now an essential part of the learning process. On the final day for medical students for example, we have a patient with a gastro-intestinal bleed who is vomiting blood. All students are asked to do is give him fluid, contact their seniors, and obtain some blood. F1s (a year ahead) meet the same patient but now they have to match the patient's blood, because when it arrives they need to know it's the wrong blood group. When they come back as F2s it is exactly the same patient but sitting

next to him is an SP who says 'You can't give this man blood, he's a Jehovah's Witness.' How do they respond? At this point they need to know they can only act on the available written evidence.

According to the nature of the role, we prepare SPs with a series of key points. For example: be prepared to be very upset if the doctor says 'x' or 'y'; never say you have a document you cannot produce. Begin by being very compliant and agreeable, but become steadily more assertive and determined; register the detail of how the doctor talks to you and be prepared to describe it in lay language.

SPs can contribute to a debrief by providing faculty members with feedback on how they felt. They may do this in character. And a skilled SP may be given the opportunity to re-run or continue discussions as part of the debrief in a 'fishbowl' format.

Assumption One – *it's all about levels*

We start with and remain sensitive to where the learners are and where it is appropriate for them be at the end of the day. At one level we assume all adult learners will have different starting points, but additionally we have to be as sensitive to where they are in their professional training and where they are in regard to simulated learning opportunities. I like to think of our approach in terms of *immersion simulation*.

For a Core Medical Training (CMT) course in the advanced simulation centre we provide our candidates with a near realistic environment. This demands that doctors and nurses engage with 'patients' in 'real time'. That puts the patient on the bed in a context that demands engagement in a natural way. Turning round from the bed, you don't see a row of colleagues watching you struggle; you see the ward and the drug cabinet and the nurse. There is no escape from the reality of the thing and they are immersed in the moment and the place. There would be no such expectation on an Advanced Life Support (ALS) course for which the manikin can be used anywhere.

Much depends on how we set things up. So the moment a CMT doctor steps through the scenario door is the moment that tests the effectiveness of our spade work. We want them to stay in role. We don't care whether they are as stressed as they might be at work when struggling to save a sick patient; or whether they are stressed because the sick patient whose recovery they are trying to bring about is a manikin and because they are being filmed and watched by their peers. **What we care about is that the circumstances and nature of the scenario enable them to be themselves, living a real life at that moment.** So, when they snap at the nurse or ignore the patient we know that's genuine behaviour from which they can learn.

Assumption Two – *everything comes back to the quality of facilitation.*

Facilitation requires a high level of concentration, focus on learning imperatives, and attention to each participant's performance. The effort to sustain this all day is considerable; and frequently it is every day. Sometimes the technology provides the problem. There is a glass screen, a one-way mirror, and we have a video feed. It's important that observers can hear and see everything clearly, including both sides of any phone conversations. Manikin technology still has a long way to go. They have little microphones in their chests that can be over-ridden by all the creaks and whirrs coming from the plastic rubbing together. From the control room, we are able to watch and listen to the medical students in the seminar-viewing room. They get so engaged with what's happening in the 'sim' room they shout at the participants. They think they know what is wrong with the patient; they can see it

all; they think they can predict what action is needed. Simulation offers unique opportunities to provide objective feedback: there are losses due to not having a genuine clinical interaction with a real patient but there are advantages too. 'When you were ventilating the patient the oxygen concentration in his lungs was AB%; when an expert anaesthetist does this they can get CD%; the average for all learners of your grade last year was EF%'

Action in the 'sim' room is sandwiched between the briefing and the debriefing, both an essential element of facilitation. This is action learning with an underlying assumption that learners are responsible for their own reflective learning. During the debrief we have the opportunity to add value based on what we've witnessed – if we remember – and alighting on opportune points while the group discusses the recordings. Facilitation for us is thus part organizational and part interactive.

Training faculty – *look at what's happening as if it is a black box*

The faculty team changes constantly as hospital staff find time to join us. Unfortunately, the pace of work and changeover of staff leaves little opportunity for formal training. To new faculty members we say, 'Think of a day course as a machine, watch it running as if it is a black box and just try to fit in with that'. Then, when you understand how it all works, you can start to manipulate the black box. You can focus on what your role is in relationship with the learner. There is the matter of identifying the intellectual, clinical discipline in order to challenge learners during the scenario, as it unfolds. Initially, there is a tendency to give what I call 'an amateur performance'. For example if you give the new colleague the role of patient (the voice of the manikin) and the doctor comes in and says 'Hello I'm Dr Jones' and the patient says 'Hello doctor, I've got crushing central chest pain radiating into my jaw and going down my left arm, I think it's my heart'. That's not what we need. We need the new colleague to respond as the patient with his or her slant on the symptoms.

Key to healthcare simulation is an understanding that the creation of learning opportunities requires faculty teams to be honest but not helpful in the control room, the 'sim' room and the viewing-seminar room. In the 'sim' room, if you are playing the role of a minor team member, you cannot take over and run the event even if in real life you might. Neither must you lie or trick the learners unless there is a prepared learning objective that ensures learners will not feel unfairly tricked. In the control room we mustn't feed answers if the questions haven't been asked. In the debrief we avoid making generous judgements. 'I thought you did really well' is an opinion with little learning value. A faculty member with more experience will respond realistically to questions while taking note of how the interview is going – the interpersonal skills the learner is exhibiting. More experience helps in the invention of verbal challenges from the patient (Am I going to die?) rather than working from an outline script or brief.

Occasionally, we see neon 'light-bulbs' going on, though it's not every day. We try to capture those moments and learn from them as well as from the subtler cues from more subdued light-bulb moments. Our emotional intelligence has to work really hard to build insights over the course of the day. For new faculty, part of what you say to them is that there are as many means to provide challenges within each scenario as there are to provide challenges and support during the debrief. If you build up those skills it is almost impossible to make an irretrievable mistake, providing you're honest and constructive and credible.

Sustaining commitment – *it's been a learning journey for us*

When we started in 2004 we knew we needed to learn – this was one of our targets. We were aware that there was a difference between competence and performance. That was really where we began. So it's been a journey for us as well. In those early days we used quite simple strategies for medical students. We studied tools such as communication loops and sharing mental models. This involved moving on from just standing in front of the patient and screaming to the heavens 'I need some oxygen', to saying *'Nurse Jones would you be so kind as to get some oxygen and put it on this patient, he is very hypoxic. Will you then come back and let me know when that has been done'.* That was about as clever as we got. Now we've learned barrels of stuff about human factors and behaviour and communication strategies. We are now providing a more learner-safe, tailor-made package because of our skill at observing what's happening and being able to turn that into credible messages for new faculty members.

I came to this job by way of a science degree. I have an MSc in Chemical Spectroscopy and worked as a Senior Operating Department Practitioner, a member of the Operating Theatre team. Anything but a standard career progression! Over time I've become hypersensitive to the fact that I must be situationally aware, to have a helicopter view, all the time. Beyond that, I've often asked myself what sustains the commitment and the concentration. Working with new faculty members from different specialties helps, but I think feedback at the debriefing is a key factor. We work so hard as a faculty team to support groups through the day that, to be frank, they would find it hard to be nasty or too critical. Watching them learn, I build a picture. Among the twelve medical students in an arc in front of us, there is the anxious one, there is the arrogant so-and-so who knows everything, the one who really wants to do well, and occasionally the one who doesn't believe in simulation. I'm aware of the different tools I've used with each of them while, at the same time, a lot of what I do happens on autopilot. Each day is unique. Therein lies the passion and hopefully, the achievement. I go home convinced (still too much on my own internal validation) that there is no better (no more enjoyable) way to spend a day that will deliver more learning about clinical performance and human behaviour with its impact upon patient safety. I'm assured in the knowledge that we usually achieve a high optimal learning level.

Andy Buttery is Specialist Trainer at Trent Simulation and Clinical Skills Centre, Nottingham University NHS Hospitals Trust

Ten

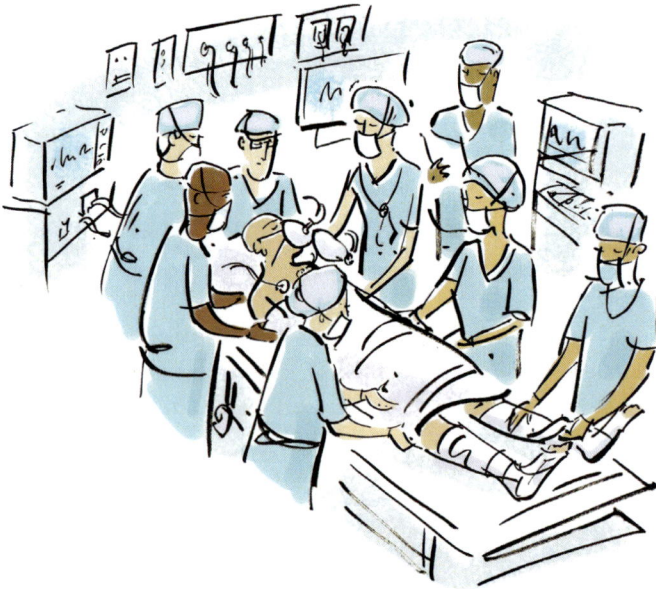

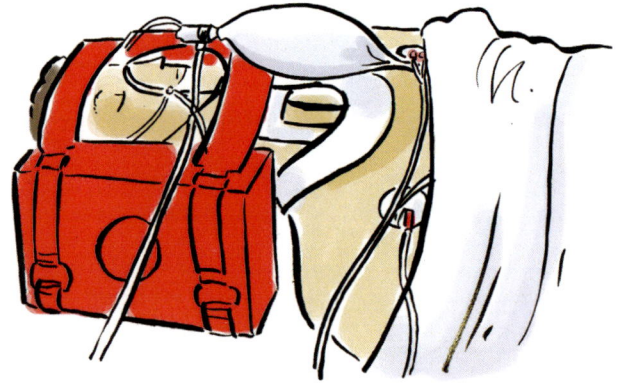

Simulated Patients in Emergency Medicine

Interview with Frank Coffey

From what I understand, the work you've been developing with SPs charts a unique pathway between the customary high and low tech areas of the SP simulation spectrum, but let's put that aside for the moment and start by looking at how you became interested in simulation, as an emergency medicine specialist.

I first came across simulated patients in the early 1990s, when as a junior doctor newly arrived from Ireland, I was asked to do an Acute Trauma Life Support Course (ATLS). This course is sponsored by the American College of Surgeons, but devised by a doctor, who, after experiencing the inability of a local hospital to help him and his relatives survive an air crash, decided something had to change. The course has the customary knowledge-based lectures and skill-stations supplemented, to my surprise, by simulations of trauma patients. They have realistic looking wounds and injuries done with theatrical make-up – moulage, as we now call it. I vividly recall this experience triggering the same emotions I have in resuscitation rooms with multiple-injury patients. Certainly more real than any training I'd previously done with manikins. That's what set me going.

I became convinced that simulation is applicable, whether for medically acute conditions like breathlessness, or for traumatic conditions, like a fracture. These kinds of conditions, including altered sensation or weakness are all very amenable to simulation.

My next experience was as an examiner for the College of Emergency Medicine, when I became involved in writing some of their original clinical OSCEs. The College was using actors at the time. I well remember observing one of these exams and watching an actor present with a cartilage knee injury. He'd had little training, just been told where to say 'ouch' and how to move his leg. It was easy to imagine how a candidate, having failed that part of the OSCE, could come back to complain about the unfair lack of authenticity. That sparked my interest in simulating complex

Levels	Symptoms	Physical Signs	Emotional Complexity	Simulation Skills	Feedback/Assessment
5	Able to assess history taking in high stakes situations.	Able to asses physical signs in high stakes situations.			Able to train other SPs to assess and choose SPs for assessment.
4	Depth/breadth of knowledge Ability to teach.	Depth/breadth of knowledge Underpinning signs Ability to teach underpinning signs. Ability to teach.	Depth of knowledge Flexibility within role Ability to teach communication	High level simulation skills. Focus Masking Consistency	Understands context of assessment in more depth including organisational/ institutional requirements. communication.
3	More complex symptoms. Ability to contextualise history. Can interpret complex scripts Give formative feedback.	Complex or multiple signs e.g. stroke, pneumothorax. Complex make-up. Formative feedback	Complex behaviour influenced by personality, culture, experience. Formative feedback		Understands key concepts and principles. Uses feedback and questioning effectively. Formative feedback.
2	Two or more symptoms. Some understanding	More specific signs , e.g. appendicitis. Simple make-up		Can simulate realistically. Able to portray realistically – pain, anger, fear	Pendleton's rules
1	Simple, e.g. sore throat.	Gross signs, e.g. tenderness of thigh	Basic behaviour patterns, e.g. fear, anger	Simple mimicry/ simulation. Minimal emotion.	Simple – "I would like that student as my doctor"
0		None	Simple interpersonal responses.		None

physical signs as well as identifying different levels of SP competence. It led me on to design an Open College Network accredited module course with New College, Nottingham, where we taught volunteers to simulate 'physical signs' for assessment. It was a pilot module. Though it never went further than that, **the chart above illustrates what I was trying to do.**

We involved professional actors, health-care workers or friends of friends as simulators for the course. A real mix of people! At the time we were lucky to have an experienced simulated patient to help with training. Unfortunately, because I wasn't directly involved in teaching at the time, these people were never used. However, there was already a parallel group of volunteer simulators working in the medical school whose purpose was basic history taking and physical examination – I think they were there for their bodies!

You've mentioned simulating physical signs which sounds rather specialised to me – do you mind explaining what it involves?

Let's begin with a medical distinction: a symptom is what a patient complains of and a sign is what a clinician finds on examination, either by observation, palpation or by testing for sensation. For instance, you can simulate a ligament knee sprain, radial palsy, shoulder injuries, or heart attacks with pain, along with the associated nausea. Another example would be a collapsed lung, a pneumothorax – for which an SP can look as if she's breathing without moving the right side of her chest. In America, their SPs simulate a thyroid bruie, by making the noise you hear as a result of the increased blood flowing through the thyroid. Neurological signs such as pain and tenderness are easy to do. There are other examples, though it is not possible to simulate sweating or blue lips.

Replicating these signs can be difficult for SPs. For example, if they are to simulate the tenderness around a ligament sprain of the knee, SPs need to know the clinician's system of examination. Unless the SP knows how the clinician will be testing for tenderness and pain it's possible they will indicate the wrong side of the knee and thereby lose their credibility. Similar problems exist with radial nerve injuries when some movements with your fingers are possible but others not. It's a bit like putting your hand out to have your blood pressure taken for a student nurse. If you've never had it taken before, you wouldn't know you need to do that. SPs have to be aware of these pitfalls. Replicating these signs can also be difficult for SP trainers who, if not clinicians, have to be limited to neurological examinations.

Thank you. What did you do next?

Soon afterwards, I became involved with a masters level degree course developed for GP trainers and hospital doctors for which we used simulated patients. In addition, and more integral to my intention of incorporating simulation into everyday practice, is the four-week attachment for medical students so they can gain experience of dealing with very sick patients, team work and the associated interpersonal skills. For this they spend two weeks in the emergency department and two weeks in anaesthetics in any one of the different trusts under the university umbrella. I lead the Nottingham University Hospitals NHS Trust component. For this we try to develop simulation exercises around multiple trauma and acutely injured patients. In support we have a training course in acute injuries and multiple-trauma, with the help of a cohort of SPs now affiliated to the emergency department.

Much of the above is either for students or off-the-job training but I'm aware that you are deeply involved in on-the-job training. How is that managed?

First, I need to explain the many constraints affecting our team training. Some issues are clinical and others organisational. For example, though it's not difficult to teach knee examinations with scant attention to the patient attached to the knee – we've done that too often – we've separated communication from the clinical skills, so that's a constant sub-text. More critically, our nurses don't get any on-going education, so they get thrown, ill prepared, into complex simulation scenarios. So there is an issue about their medical knowledge. If they join the emergency department they'll get an induction for a week and that's it. Whereas, historically there used to be senior nurses on the shop floor teaching them – now those senior nurses currently in the NHS are running around chasing targets. As a result, the nurses who don't have an appropriate level of clinical knowledge feel very vulnerable and exposed.

The organisational issues concern changing practice and time to train. Whereas, previously there was a lot of training in the old specialty 'firm' structure, clinicians now inevitably work, even more so, as independent practitioners. They have their job rotas and they do their nine clinical sessions together with one SPA (Supporting Professional Activities) of four hours for their necessary management catch-ups. There is very limited capacity for training. It's the same for facilitator training. It's crucial for facilitators to know a patient's actual pulse is not the pulse the monitor is recording, to give just one example. And that's why we're now trying to generate our own income so we can deliver courses within the emergency department to develop the whole institution's expertise.

To that end we now have our own teaching fellow and clinical educators, and the present cohort of SPs, who will become part of the department's educational infrastructure. At present there are 14 SPs which we'd like to expand to 40 for use on a daily basis for multi-professional education, i.e. team training at all levels within the department. We still have to win over the nursing educators – nurses do seem to struggle with simulation, so we need nurse facilitators to manage change on that front. I'm doing all this in spite of… well it's a passion. The two biggest problems that prevent us realising our vision are simulation facilitation and current nursing practice.

While I can appreciate the institutional problems you face, the trauma team building scenario I witnessed came over as powerful simulated training

The answer to that is, 'yes – but'. There is a specific problem with multiple-trauma and possibly other acute scenarios. People have fixed roles for multiple-trauma that don't apply in other team situations. There is nurse one, nurse two and nurse three who should each have clearly defined roles. Previously there has been no fuller team training, so the first issue has been these role definitions. Easily said, but that depends on how the different roles and their team leaders operate. Should there be a nurse leader, for example? Having got the roles sorted out you then need a buy-in from the team leaders. You can do all the training in the world but if you come to a real situation and no one has bought into the methodology you might as well forget it. That is what happened a couple of years ago. We had about £7000 to spend. So we designed the team roles and went over to the Sim Centre where every nurse in the department practised the methodology with the manikin. When they came back it had all gone out of the window, largely because of lack of senior consultant buy in. We tried to make it as real as possible but with manikins you do tend to lose the reality, particularly if people are not convinced of the training need in the first place.

There must be light at the end of the tunnel?

Well we intend training to be as real as possible, that includes understanding the nature of a changing workplace. We will soon have a new department where patients will be admitted medically with a nurse-led discharge unit for

patients in for short stay observation. We have also run a ten week course in moulage, so going back to my early ATLS experience, we can now have a live person with realistic wounds moaning and groaning – what more would you want!

We've talked around the trauma team training scenario, could we now look at it in detail – how does it work?

Each training episode starts with a briefing: identifying the roles, testing out how they work, deciding if they need tweaking and how they'll happen role-wise. During the briefing the final touches are made to the moulage wounds. It then starts in the reality of a working emergency department. The paramedics arrive with the patient, who has a ruptured spleen and is in shock because of the bleeding. The team are all there for the handover – with all the roles in place, including a waiting consultant. The handover details are recorded on a board which all the team can see as they are subsequently amended. The patient is examined – an examination that combines patient responses and moulage evidence of bruising and wounds. With medical students on their critical illness days we can 'time out' if they get really flummoxed, but this is real, so real you can hear other cases coming and going elsewhere in the department. I experienced just how real it has become when I wandered in and stood by the trolley without being noticed. Everyone just carried on. Moreover, one of the consultants playing a role was actually on call when a cardiac arrest was brought in. The team leader who tried to drag him in to review the abdomen in the trauma simulation thought he was simulating when he said he had to go. In the early days this might have been the case but now we've agreed we need a code word – it's 'no duff'. The simulation finishes when the patient is wheeled off for the next stage of treatment. We then retire for the debrief.

The value of the debrief is twofold: it enables personal learning, (always on the assumption that decisions will be incorporated in future action), and as important for me, that I can adjust the effectiveness of any future training. Having a living and breathing SP is essential. We've now done five or six of these full-scale training events for which the resource input is massive – a different take on *facilitation* with its organisational demands. There's the setting up: sorting out the moulage, training the SP, fitting up the hybrid stuff with the intravenous access and the bloods, attaching the drip, timetabling staff availability, to mention a few issues. Only twice have we been able to do this in situ. Other episodes have taken place in the non-operational clinical skill area. The overriding question of how to spread training to the whole department remains. Needless to say, I'm still optimistic!

Dr Frank Coffey is Consultant in Emergency Medicine (EM) and EM Lead DREEAM (Department of Research and Education in Emergency medicine Acute medicine and Major trauma), Nottingham University NHS Hospitals Trust. He is also an Associate Professor at the University of Nottingham Medical School and Professor/Academic in Residence, Royal College of Surgeons in Ireland.

Eleven

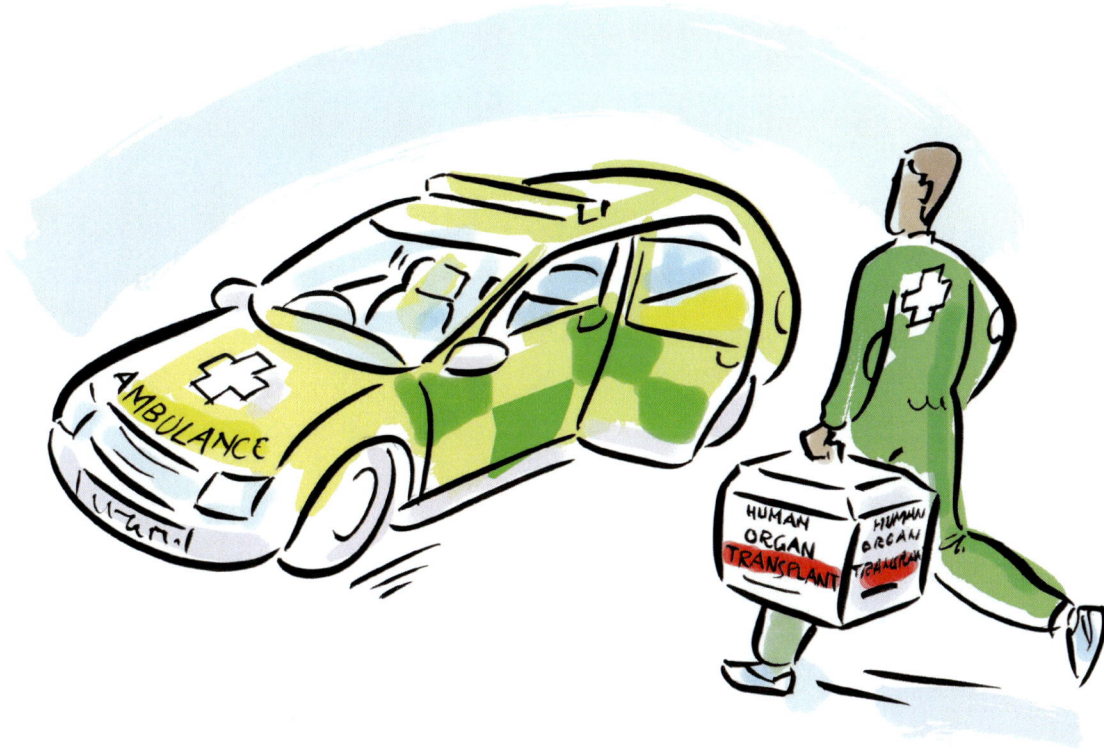

Deceased Donation Simulation

Dale Gardiner

Origins of the course

The Organ Donor Task Force (2008) asked every hospital Trust/Board in the UK to nominate a clinical lead for organ donation (CLOD) together with the establishment of an organ donation committee chaired by a non-clinician. When I became CLOD for Nottingham University Hospitals the priority was a clearer organ donation pathway, particularly for Donation after Circulatory Death.

To be effective, this necessitated a whole hospital approach, no easy task because it must include several clinical specialties. I was also sensitive to the fact that my colleagues in Adult Intensive Care and other specialties were not getting exposure to good cross-hospital practice. Organ donation is inevitably emotionally fraught. What was needed then, and still is, is a course that follows the patient's journey across various specialisms, at the same time as rehearsing the challenging conversations that must be held with relatives of the dying and deceased potential donor.

Using simulation, we needed to create a realistic, immersive environment in which all clinical participants (faculty) can do their *own* jobs, with simulators playing the family members. Trent Simulation & Clinical Skills Centre provides a suitable on-campus venue. It has a range of accommodation and facilities to fit both the stage-by-stage clinical procedures and quiet family discussions. Observers can witness every activity on video in their adjacent debriefing room.

We submitted a business case for a pilot Multidisciplinary Training Day Simulation Course that 'mimics real life patient journeys. It begins in the emergency department (ED), leads to the recognition that death is imminent and allows for recognition and implementation of deceased donation pathways'. Only one such course had been run previously in the UK. The complexity of getting the course together will be understood if I tell you that it involves clinicians and nurses from Intensive Care, Paediatric Intensive Care, Neurosurgery (medical only) Theatre and Anaesthesia as well as the Emergency Department. Very few simulations run a patient journey where you get to see how everyone's role dovetails. Organ donation requires a whole hospital approach. It's probably the most complicated operation the NHS ever does in a single 24 hour period. The required financial support came from the Trust Organ Donation Committee, using monies given to the Trust to support Organ Donation, by NHSBT, for every consented deceased organ donor.

Course presentation

During the day, the participants and observers meet in two patient journeys. One case follows a head injury leading, over two days, to a decision to withdraw life-sustaining treatment after circulatory death and then to donation. The other follows a donation after brainstem death. Each case moves through the required hospital stages with clinical procedures taking place around the manikin patient in the 'sim' room and early conversation with relatives in a quiet room. The 'sim' room is equipped with telephones so advice can be received from consultants elsewhere in the hospital. I share the organisational aspects with two nurses who make sure faculty are in the right place with relevant paperwork at the right time, and the simulation staff. There are always many more observers than participants. Some of the clinical observers act as faculty, particularly for telephone conversations from the sim room. Because the observers watch everything that happens on video, their feedback and questions make a vital contribution at the debrief.

Observers include clinicians, NHS administrators, academics, media representatives (we've tried to get the BBC in) and coroners.

We've prepared a very detailed hand-out which guides participants and observers through the day. It includes a checklist of OD procedure suggestions regarding interpersonal skills and behaviours. Particularly relevant for such stressful meetings is an aid-list to help read relatives' non-verbal behaviours.

Learning purpose

A distinctive feature of the course, unlike what happens with junior doctor training, is that we do not correct communication or clinical behaviours – with exceptions that I will mention later. **Our purpose is to change attitudes,** cultural or otherwise. For instance, when a patient comes into the emergency department, we assume all the doctors will do the resuscitation if it is needed. We don't correct any of that. We are not interested in that! The key moment for that episode is when the relatives walk in, as happens frequently in emergency departments. Suddenly the relatives are there by the bedside. That's the bit where we want our participants to react naturally. We certainly don't want them to raise organ donation at an inappropriate moment.

As faculty we are always learning how to manage the course more effectively, sometimes over specific details. For example, we've been concerned about the appropriate time to introduce the SN-OD (Specialist Nurse Organ Donation). You can involve the SN-OD as a standard member of the team talking with relatives. Later, when the relatives find out she is concerned with organ donation, they think they're being conned. That's why we have been leaving the decision regarding SN-OD's entry to the OD process to whole group consensus. The best time to do this is emerging from collective course-on-course decisions.

More generally, **the overall purpose is to achieve an understanding of the whole process**, particularly so for the coroner or the chair of the OD committee who are non-medics.

As I mentioned, there is one bit of clinical training we give about brain-death testing and withdrawal of life-sustaining treatment with the manikin. This is to avoid a possible confusion of signs resulting from use of the manikin – it can't replicate everything a real person does! A manikin with a cough is always a bit funny.

Extract from SP Instructions

Simulator Brief – Communication 4

It is the next morning. Overnight things have worsened and you have been told Michael's (grandson) brain has become less reactive. You have tried to get some rest at home. You have returned to the hospital, as instructed the night before, to arrive after the morning ward round. It is now 10 am

- The medical team is going to talk to you again. You fear the worst.
- You will be told that Michael is not going to survive. In the course of this discussion, deceased organ donation will 'hopefully' be raised with you.
- We want you to react positively to the suggestion of organ donation, as helping others is the kind of person Michael is. He may have watched a documentary about organ donation and said it was something he would do. You don't know if he is on the organ donation register.

Questions you might ask to help participants if they don't raise donation

'What happens now?' (when told he is going to die) 'Do you just turn the machines off?' 'Which organs can be donated?'

SP involvement

'To a simulator the brief reads as a series of cues within a very clear series of episodes. At no point am I told what to say but the suggestions are indicative. This tells me that I am being trusted to act naturally. It also tells me that, though my presence is important, it is the story of the day rather than the 'how' of what happens between me/us and the people talking to us that is really important. It is what we say, not necessarily the manner of it that is crucial'. We are to be there and portray emotion – a mainly non-verbal task.
SP - EBW

We want people to act naturally, which is always hard to do in a best practice situation. So we don't want simulators who get weepy or throw themselves on the floor, or do anger! It's hard enough to talk about brain death! And that kind of behaviour is rare in these circumstances. It's not what this course is about. Our intention is to model best practice not correct behaviour. So we want the simulators to act naturally, as they would themselves, faced with this kind of situation.

Sequence of Events for Scenario One

1. **Emergency Department - 16 year old patient with isolated head injury arrives**

   Present
   EM registrar and EM nurse
   ED resuscitation area

2. **Simulated multi-disciplinary resuscitation**

   Present
   EM registrar, EM nurse, Anaesthetist
   Phone
   ED consultant and Neurosurgery consultant

3. **Family arrive at bedside**
   2 X SPs

Debrief

1. **Review CT scan**

   Present
   EM registrar & nurse, Anaesthetic & Neurosurgery registrars
   Phone
   Neurosurgery consultant

2. **Family update - Quiet room (video linked)**

   Present
   2 X SPs, Participants to decide who best to speak with SPs

Much Later

3. **Paediatric Intensive Care Unit (PICU) at bedside**

   Present
   2 X SPs, IC registrar, IC nurse

Debrief

Next Morning

1. **Overnight deterioration – possible withdrawal of treatment**

   Present
   Neurosurgery registrar, IC registrar IC nurse, 2 X SPs
   Phone
   PICU consultant, Neurosurgery consultant

2. **Referral for possible deceased donation**

   Present
   as above + Senior Nurse Organ Donation (SN-OD)

3. **Family update**
   2 X SPs
   Discuss treatment withdrawal and OD

   Present
   Participants to decide who best,
   SN-OD will request

Debrief

Hours Later

1. **Deceased lung donation agreed**
   Family present – withdrawal agreed

   Present
   IC registrar, IC nurse, 2 X SPs, SN-OD

2. **Real time from above - Lung re-intubated, lung re-inflation DCD donation**

   Present
   Anaesthetic registrar, IC registrar, SN-OD

Debrief

Debriefs

Our debrief sessions are at a much higher level than normal. Bear in mind that we are considering issues of a surgical, ethical, legal, organisational and emotional kind, altogether, at moments of tension. By doing it this way we are trying to change attitudes and explore concepts; for instance, what's happening in relatives' minds when they watch the resuscitation. It's a much higher level than anything in my experience when we have such a broad range of practitioners, all sharing their knowledge and what they've gained from taking part. That's a real strength. We have been asked who our target is – the participants, the faculty, or the observers. It seems as if I'm targeting all of them. And that's quite true. Though we don't put consultants into the simulation, they do 'pop-in' as observers, so they can 'watch their juniors'!

In the debrief, we explore use of words like death and explanations of brain death and their impact – the interaction with relatives. We explore the big themes as dictated by the scenarios.

Conducting the debrief is the nearest we get to standard facilitation. Otherwise it's a question of organisation; making sure each episode proceeds on time, in the right place with the appropriate kit.

There are two audiences for the debrief: the participants and the observers – all important for organ donation. This is as close as we can ever get them to the real thing.

Outcomes*

A lot of people say it's one of the best courses they have done. The first aspect they highlight is the senior status of the multi-disciplined practitioners; the second is that you see the whole hospital process. People say it will alter their practice but we don't have a longer term follow up. It's hard to say if it's increased organ donation numbers. There are many other factors at play.

Has it resulted in behaviour change? That's difficult to say, though surveying past participants to see if they still rate the course as well as they did say 18 months later might well be helpful.

*The results of pre- and post-questionnaire responses for the first two donation simulation days are recorded in Evaluation of deceased donation simulation, Wood, Buss, Buttery, Gardiner. *Journal of the Intensive Care Society*, Vol 13, No 2, April 2012

Dr Dale Gardiner is Intensive Care Consultant and Clinical Lead for Organ Donation at Queens Medical Centre, University of Nottingham Hospitals NHS Trust

Twelve

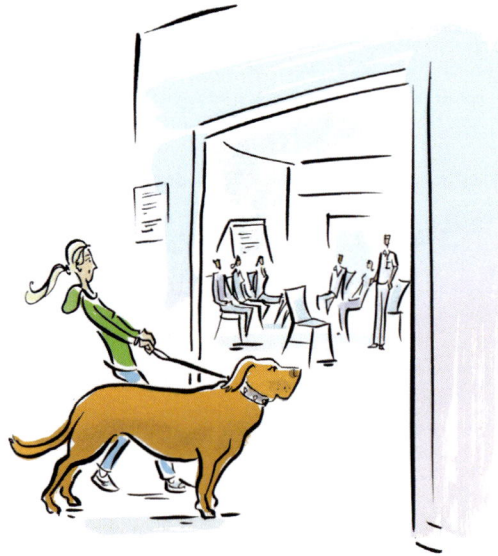

Talking with Clients – Training with SPs

University of Nottingham School of Veterinary Medicine and Science

Liz Mossop

We started using SPs to practise communicating with clients soon after the inauguration of this new, and only the seventh, Veterinary School in the UK (Dublin also has a vet school). I was receptive to the idea. I'd become interested in education as a response to teaching veterinary nurses at a previous practice. My remit here is concerned with professional skills in the widest sense: communication skills, business and management, ethics, human/animal bond, research skills, learning skills – all important in the curriculum. I discovered that SP work was already embedded in other vet schools' curricula. The veterinary communication skills movement started at Liverpool vet school in the early 2000s, where they realised that teaching was needed – the VDS (Veterinary Defence Society) knew that lots of claims against vets were due to poor communication skills and that something needed to be done. VDS funded a lecturer's position at

Liverpool, and work had already begun there to adapt the Calgary-Cambridge (C-C) guide to the veterinary context. Fortunately, they had direct contact with Jonathan Silverman and Julie Draper, the authors. As a result a custom built C-C model was published for the veterinary context. Carol Gray became the first lecturer in Veterinary Communication skills at Liverpool and began to embed communication skills within their curriculum. The NUAVCS group (National Unit for the Advancement of Veterinary Communication Skills) was also created formally. This is a network for communication skills leaders from each of the vet schools who used to meet twice a year to support each other. The network still exists and allows us to meet to train each other as facilitators or to share ideas – we now have an on-line way of meeting rather than face to face. For example, all our client scenarios are shared on a Google site.

We want our students to learn experientially; first how to take a history – in third year they do explanation and planning and in the fourth year they do a whole interview, but with difficult client situations. In the fifth year they also do complete interviews, but in a workplace context. We thus break client communication into chunks with a year-on-year sequence. Interestingly, in the second year it's become clear that you don't need any clinical knowledge to take a good history; that's after we've taught them a bit of theory about open and closed questions and that sort of thing in the first year. We have a 'client contact day', in year one when we get real clients, with real animals, so students get a chance to talk to owners. This raises the question of how they should dress and present themselves when talking with clients. Of all the teaching I do, communication skills sessions get the most positive feedback.

Students like using simulators, though some get scared. I have only ever had one student come to me and say 'I am not doing it'. My reply was, 'it's up to you – you will have an OSCE at the end of the year and you will have to do it' – so she did and with plenty of support she was fine. We've become practiced at dealing with this – fear of the unknown is the usual cause.

There can be some tension regarding this mode of learning, because it is a very different learning approach. To be fair, some tutors are more accustomed to traditional methods of delivery and see communication skill teaching as an irrelevance. We rely on trained simulators and that's an expense, but it's in the budget. And more fortunately, colleagues have come to know that students love it and learn a lot from it. It's become a very important aspect of our curriculum.

In the final year of teaching, students spend all their time on workplace rotations. So, they are communicating for real – both with colleagues and clients. However, we still wanted to deliver a more intense and controllable communication skill session in context. To that end we've developed a simulation day at Nottingham Trent University where they train veterinary nurses. They have a fabulous mock practice where we spend a day with a mixture of vet and vet nursing students, running the practice and dealing with everything from phone calls through to difficult clients at reception. This is a powerful learning experience which really teaches them to work competently with their colleagues, using each other's skill sets.

The SP resourced course

The SPs receive their scenarios before they come here. We have a briefing session so they can check out the detailed way they've personalised the case and more importantly, acquire crucial background information; very necessary, for example, with commercial as distinct from domestic clients with less familiar backgrounds for the SPs. They will then wait outside a room to be called in. Meanwhile, the group facilitators are introducing the Calgary-Cambridge framework and allocating tasks to the observers. The volunteer student then calls in the client for the interview. This is followed by observer and facilitator feedback. The SP then moves on to the next room, so each group will experience seven or so cases at 40 minute intervals, with a break – and most students in the group will have direct experience in the chair. However, the quality of the experience depends significantly upon the facilitator – which is why we train all our facilitators specifically for this type of teaching.

Communication Skills Curriculum

Year 2 History taking
Year 3 Giving information & BBN
Year 4 Difficult situations
Year 5 Simulated practice + recordings

- The simulated practice with SP clients, veterinary nurses and student involves the running of a normal vets practice.
- Students are encouraged to record themselves doing a consultation, with consent from the client. They have a template to guide their own reflective feedback.

Scenario Example - Reggie Jay

Owner: *Mr/Mrs Jay*

Animal: *Reggie, 13 year old cross breed dog, black and tan*

History: *Reggie has been under treatment at the practice for chronic liver failure for a year now. He first became ill last year with vomiting and lethargy. Initially symptomatic treatment (anti-sickness injection and light diet) were prescribed, but when he got no better the vet advised blood tests. These test showed severe liver disease and he also became jaundiced quite quickly. He has since been managed on some medication (tablets) and although he has been losing weight since then, he has remained reasonably happy and his appetite got slightly better. However, over the last month the weight loss has progressed and his appetite has slowly declined. He doesn't really have much interest in life and so the family have made the decision that he should now be put to sleep.*

Information for simulator: *This has been a tough decision to make due to the slow progression of Reggie's liver failure. You brought Reggie in last week to see the vet and he said that there were no more treatment options. You went home to discuss this with the family. You have now returned to speak to the receptionist about making an appointment for the PTS. You want to know:*

- *Would they advise a house visit or should you bring him in?*
- *What happens during the procedure?*
- *Can you stay with him? How about your 10 year old daughter and your husband/wife?*
- *What happens afterwards – you want to know what the options are regarding the body.*

You are quite business-like at first but this is a brave face, and if the student shows empathy then you will get quite sad and upset, leave long silences. What you really need is to be asked to sit down and have a one-to-one chat with whoever deals with you as you need to talk about what a difficult decision this has been. You are really quite worried about the loss of Reggie and the effect it will have on your daughter, and would appreciate any advice. You will be very receptive to any mention of pet bereavement counselling – there is a help line they could direct you to. If they mention a book of memories or planting a tree or something similar you will also be open to this and be very grateful.

During this session a good student will:

1. *Establish a good rapport with the client by demonstrating empathy for the situation*
2. *Explain clearly all the options around euthanasia and disposal of the body*
3. *Take the client to one side to have the discussion*
4. *Offer pet bereavement options*
5. *Check for further concerns*

Facilitation

We ask facilitators to follow a framework for each client case:

1. Introduce themselves and describe the purpose of the session – framework on board?
2. Outline the scenario and organise the student interview sequence
3. Identify personal agendas for feedback purposes
4. Prepare the group – give out observation tasks
5. Run the client case session (including opportunity to 'time out')
6. Get feedback from the student in the chair
7. Observer feedback + feedback from SP, in or out of role* **then** Conduct Plenary Feedback at conclusion of the last session

For some of these sessions we do make recordings, although this can have a diverting influence on students!

I am dictatorial about feedback. There are two rules:

- **You cannot give feedback unless you record what you see.**
- **If you say that was good – I want an example**

Student frameworks. These are to be used in conjunction within the structure of the facilitator framework. For example, the history taking framework* includes:

1. Prepare yourself
2. Start with an open question
3. Move into closed questions as necessary
4. Use screening and summarising
5. Establish rapport and use empathy
6. Be aware of body language

* We make the point that frameworks are not rule books – they are there to help if you get lost.

Facilitator training

As we are a new school, we wanted as many staff as possible to become trained facilitators whether they were clinicians or not. This does mean there are differences between facilitators, and SPs often comment on this. Clearly, we need to keep the training level up. To that end we have trainers from the VDS and we help out with training at other schools to keep our skills up to date.

We are joined by SPs for the facilitator training in order to replicate the task as authentically as possible. Each participant takes a turn as facilitator and receives feedback from the group. They also have a turn at being the student which can be cathartic as we run difficult scenarios as well as difficult students. When directly engaged with students, the briefing notes provide a safety net which includes the framework structure recommended for that particular session.

However much we plan I think it can be said that these SP sessions are never less than enjoyable. Indeed, they can be life changing. Two moments stand out in my memory. First with a student – we have an excellent scenario in the simulation day run for Year 5. Students are presented with a rabbit together with a consent form that says the rabbit is to be spayed. The owner is very concerned about the procedure because it's his daughter's rabbit. The student has to do a pre-op consultation – the rabbit is real and is male. The student finishes the consultation but does not do a physical examination. Oh dear, it's not possible to spay a male rabbit!!! – a big learning moment?

The second experience I will not forget happened during training. A very experienced and probably slightly cynical member of staff who'd come for facilitator training was confronted by a very angry client. It was painful to witness how taken aback he was by the reality, which he admitted and later said was the best thing he'd done. Many of the experienced vets we've trained as facilitators report that their own consultation style has changed as a result – it's strange how this essential skill receives so little attention at postgraduate level.

Liz Mossop is Associate Professor of Veterinary Education and Sub Dean for Teaching, Learning and Assessment at University of Nottingham School of Veterinary Medicine and Science

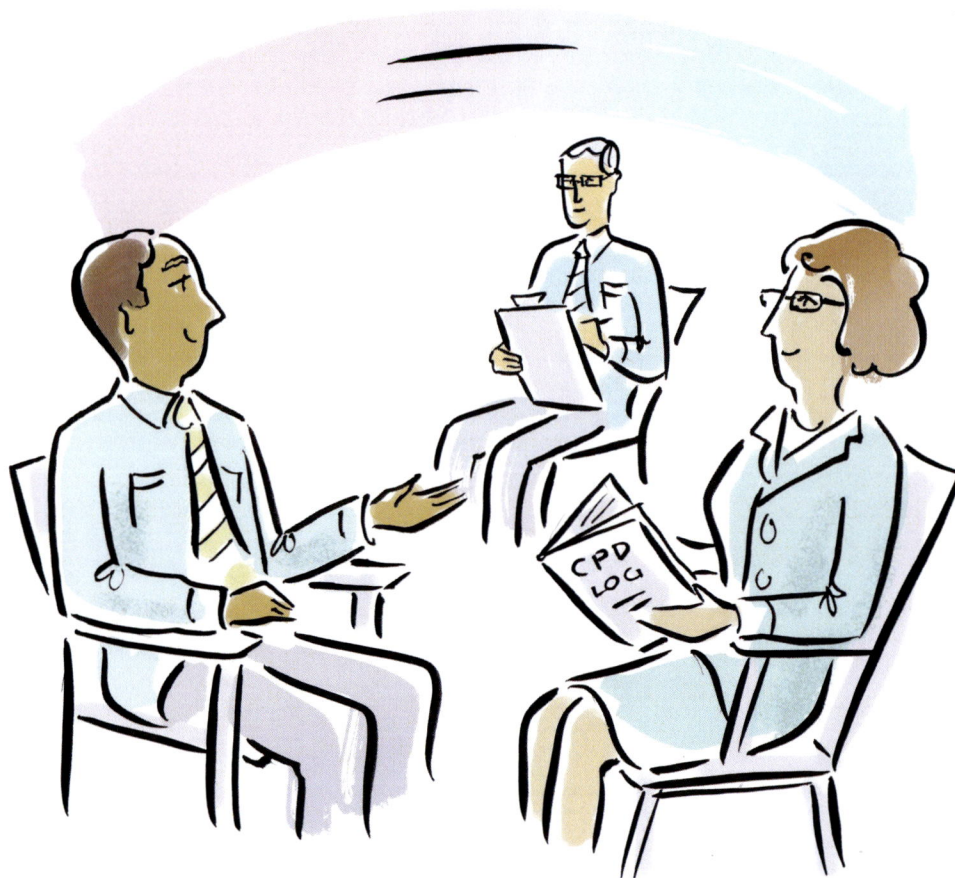

Simulating Doctors for GP Appraiser Training

Amanda Portnoy

Background to appraiser training

Annual appraisal for GPs has been in place since 2002. The process is carried out at an annual meeting between a trained GP appraiser and each GP in the region; it affords an opportunity for GPs to discuss the full scope of their work, to reflect on their ongoing learning, on how improvements might be made and to plan their learning for the ensuing year. Appraisal plays a central role in the Revalidation process which demonstrates at regular 5 yearly intervals that doctors are up to date and fit to practice.

The GMC has dictated that doctors have to collect supporting information confirming their participation in Continuing Professional Development, Quality Improvement Activity, Significant Event Analysis, Feedback from patients and colleagues and a review of any complaints or plaudits received.

The appraisal provides an opportunity for the doctor to discuss the supporting information collected over a year and reflect on it under the four GMC Good Medical Practice Domains of 'Knowledge, skills and performance', 'Safety and quality', 'Communication, partnership and teamwork' and 'Maintaining trust', e.g. in the form of case histories, teaching or further audit of their practice.

Evidence of Continuing Professional Development (CPD) is a professional responsibility and as such forms an important part of the appraisal discussion. It can encompass attendance at lectures, seminars, group discussions, reading or e-learning together with examples of reflection and actions that may follow. A course attendance certificate is considered a more valuable piece of supporting information if the doctor can relate it to changes in their practice or produce evidence of reflection in terms of application of the knowledge.

There is a wide range in the amount of energy GPs devote to the process. CPD activity varies from 50 to a carefully logged 300 hours. The standard requirement is for 50 hours with supporting evidence of reflection. It may be about ways to currently manage a condition such as hypertension or diabetes. It's not unusual for doctors to reflect internally without actually recording this, so one of the appraiser's roles is to skilfully draw this reflection out and help the doctor with ways to demonstrate it. We have about 100 appraisers for Nottingham and Derby whose task is to establish what the doctor has done and support or challenge what emerges from the interview and record this in a succinct summary under the GMC Domain headings. We have used SPs to practise how best to conduct this interview and to look at different ways to approach different scenarios.

SPs as doctors – the roles

The nature of extended professional learning and its application is the stuff of the annual interview with an appraiser. Simulators, as appraisees, need to be aware of the general requirements as well as the particular details of the doctor they represent.

SPs are used mainly for appraiser update training on half day courses. We have developed a number of different characters for our SPs to portray and they are usually run on the day with six SPs, each of whom choose one or more roles they can identify with. Beforehand, we do a run through of each character's role and the scenario we wish them to play. We also explain the various aspects of general practice they need to be aware of, including the primary care team structure, telephone consultations, home visiting arrangements and things like QOF, IT, Choose & Book and the difference between a GMS and PMS GP contract.

The SP roles we have developed cover half a side of A4 – they describe a GP of a personality type that can be a challenge to an appraiser and an appraisal situation that would potentially be difficult to deal with. To some extent the roles are stereotypical, but they do represent the extremes that appraisers might only have to deal with very rarely, but spend a lot of time worrying about! For example, one describes a young GP returning from maternity leave too early, who has symptoms of post-natal depression, which she is trying hard to push into the background. Then there is a senior doctor nearing retirement who feels he's done it all before and doesn't see the need to demonstrate his ability to an appraiser. Another scenario concerns a fast talking doctor who likes to fly by the seat of his or her pants and doesn't like to do any in-depth thinking about his education; a superficial learner. We instruct the SPs in roles playing GPs with portfolio careers: a doctor returning after a career break, the part time salaried GP role and the full time overcommitted full time GP partner, the garrulous over-confident doctor and the doctor lacking in confidence, the struggling doctor and the high flyer. We construct short summaries of mock appraisal folders of supporting information for each SP character.

Background knowledge

Whatever role the SP plays, in order to maintain their credibility, they need to be aware of some of the basic principles of being a GP and this is where the initial familiarisation sessions are of value. The supporting information appraisees bring will contain some clinical information and we need to make sure SPs know enough to discuss this in a credible way. For example if the supporting information relates to a clinical audit, they are instructed on what it is about, why it was done and a brief description of the findings. They also need to know what changes it might lead to in their practice. Doctors often get into discussions about clinical management or other aspects of medicine that the SP is not familiar with. If the interview starts to head in this direction we instruct the SPs to ask for a 'Process stop' or 'Time out' – this enables the interview to re-focus along lines more familiar to the SP. The aim of the exercise is to explore challenging situations or behaviour rather than to have an in-depth clinical debate.

The aim is for the SP to know enough to justify the learning that has taken place and its outcome. It involves keeping the interview away from areas of ignorance. On the other hand, because the roles mainly feature attitudinal problems, and the appraisers are well aware that the purpose is to explore issues of that kind, they are unlikely to pursue clinical matters in depth. There is an element of collusion with reality here.

It's different for more complex interviews, with a critical clinical focus; for which SPs would need more clinical background information. That's not impossible to provide, but whether it is economically useful to spend time on this for role play is another matter. Certainly, in scenarios concerning various complex job roles, attitudes, depression, lack of motivation, challenging behaviour, stress or team dynamics, we have found SPs convincing. Discussing clinical minutiae is more difficult to grapple with. That said, the SPs I've had contact with are good at appropriate improvisation if it is not in the script!

In action-interviews

Depending on the venue, we usually have one big room with three or four breakout rooms. Appraiser update sessions usually cater for 20/30 people at a time. Several interviews can take place in the big room at the same time, and at each there will be an appraiser, an appraisee (SP) and one or more observers. The lead observers, an experienced GP Appraiser or GP educator, will have a tick list of required appraiser competences based on the RST (Revalidation Support Team) Appraisers Competency Framework. We have an agreed process stop 'Time out' when the SP or any member of the discussion can hold a hand up if things get stuck. It's not what happens in reality, but it is valuable because the GP educator can unpack what's been happening and then say to the SP, 'Wind that back and play it differently next time'. We have found that SPs are very good at that.

It's fascinating to see how a written scenario can develop into an unpredicted tussle between doctor and appraiser.

Feedback

Good Appraiser feedback at appraisal involves active listening, empathic understanding and careful drawing out of the doctor's strengths and areas for improvement An important part of this is helping the appraisee to plan their future education. We have found SPs are good at giving objective feedback to the appraisers on how they have performed! They will say if they feel they've been helped, just as they will if they think the appraiser was on the wrong tack. SPs follow a model that demands constructive feedback and they are accustomed to expressing their feelings.

Value

SPs seem to have the ability to be outcome focused in the simulated appraisal discussion. If you give two doctors some clinical information, they can become totally engrossed in the clinical context – to the exclusion of the appraisal process – and will start discussing the management of a disease. Although interesting and valuable, this isn't what should normally take place. The appraiser needs to find out what that doctor has gained from their learning and how it is going to change their practice. SPs are less likely to go down the clinical discussion path; they'll keep the interview on an appraisal footing.

There is no reason why SPs shouldn't be used. Certainly for appraisal update training looking at problems such as the challenging behaviour scenarios mentioned earlier. These problems rarely occur but are something appraisers worry about, and it's valuable to have a rehearsal opportunity. The interpersonal skills involved are transferable to any situation so it is valuable to use SPs. For me, the problem is creating convincing role play scenarios, getting it organised and returning to the situation where we can call in a group of SPs who don't need any additional training.

It is valuable for an appraiser to be able to rehearse how they might handle difficult situations, to offer support to non-standard appraisees and to practise facilitating a well-structured and focused appraisal under difficult circumstances.

Once we had a cohort of SPs trained in the basic skills, we found they demonstrated an ability to adopt similar appraisee roles with a minimum of additional input, and this was clearly valuable in arranging subsequent training sessions.

Amanda Portnoy is a practising GP, a Locality Appraiser Lead for Nottingham and Derbyshire and an Appraiser Trainer for East Midlands Local Education and Training Board (formerly the East Midlands Deanery).

At a GP Appraisal workshop I was part of, the GP participants were clearly told that the 'under-performing peers' they'd be interacting with were simulators. My role was that of a rather arrogant, uncooperative GP who was an expert in diabetes. During the first coffee break, I was approached by the participant who'd just been appraising me. 'So … 'he said. 'Where do you practise?' It's good to know how convincing a simulation can be! SP - GG

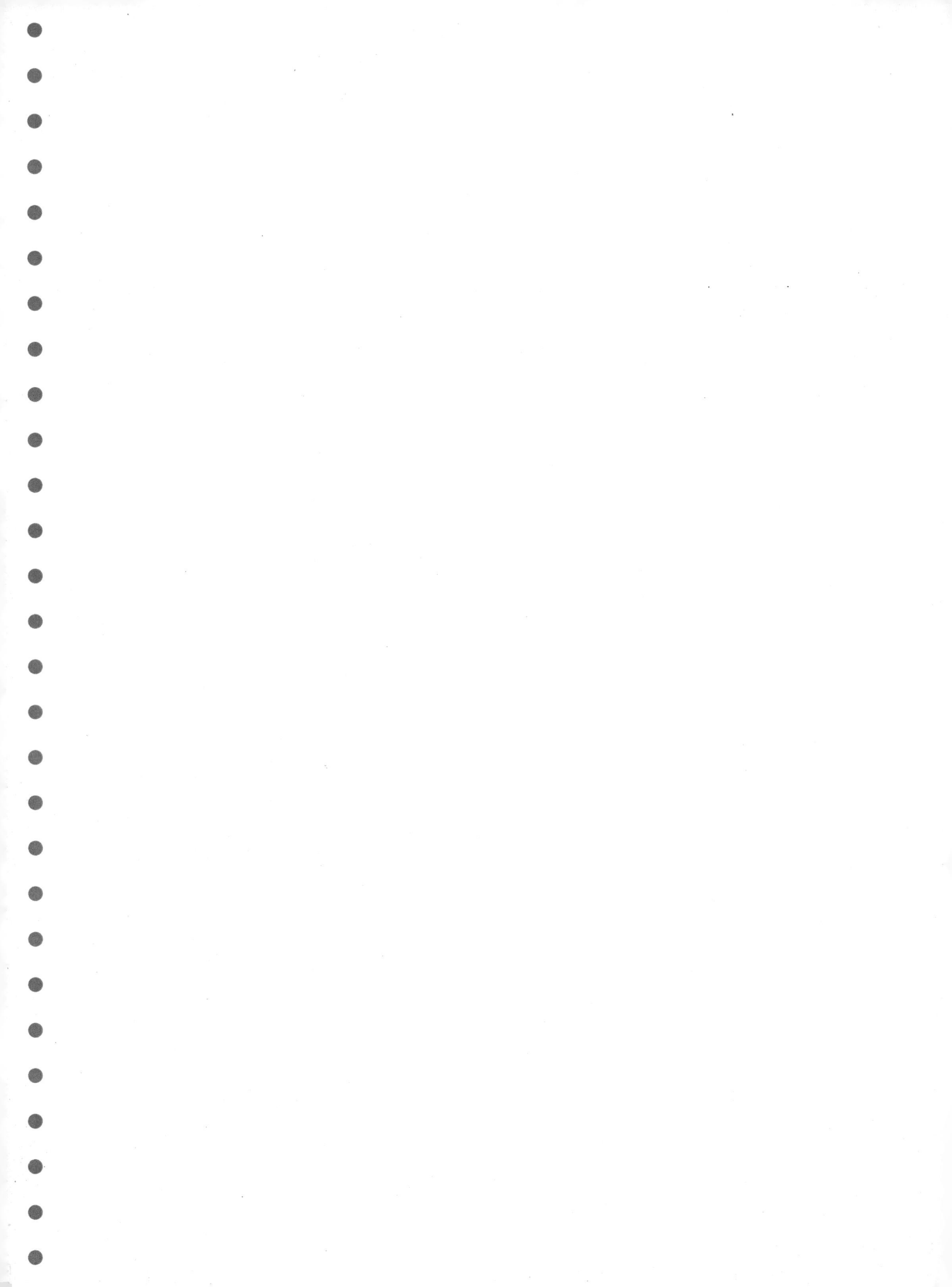